Vasectomy Reversal

Sheldon H. F. Marks

Vasectomy Reversal

Manual of Vasovasostomy
and Vasoepididymostomy

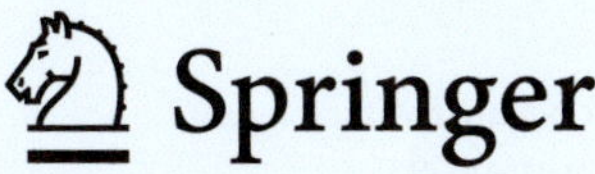 Springer

Sheldon H. F. Marks
University of Arizona College of Medicine
International Center Vasectomy Reversal
Tucson, AZ
USA

ISBN 978-3-030-13115-9   ISBN 978-3-030-00455-2   (eBook)
https://doi.org/10.1007/978-3-030-00455-2

Preface

A vasectomy reversal is one of the most rewarding yet technically challenging procedures in the urologist's armamentarium. As vasectomies continue to be one of the most common procedures in medicine, and with continued advances in microsurgical reversal techniques, combined with increased consumer awareness, the demand for reversals is increasing. Up to 6% of men who have had a vasectomy subsequently change their minds and choose a vasectomy reversal, the most cost-effective approach to fathering children after vasectomy. What is frustrating is that far too many doctors and even urologists are unaware of these new advances in microsurgical techniques and the increased success up to 99.5%.

What makes discussing the success of a vasectomy reversal especially difficult is the wide range of training, skills, and experience of the urologists that perform this surgery. In fact, the majority of reversals are performed on an occasional basis by general urologists, often using a variety of techniques learned during their training, sometimes many years to decades ago. As with every other surgical technique in medicine, advances over the years have contributed to much higher successes with fewer complications in experienced hands.

The intent of this book is to highlight many of these advances, technical points, and associated decision-making that I use when performing a state-of-the-art vasectomy reversal.

The relative paucity of data in the literature on many of these topics, rationale for techniques, and the lack of consistent definitions of endpoints drives many of these recommendations for care and technical expertise to be based primarily on expert opinion from international leaders. Because even the most experienced "reversalist" will never hit a plateau of learning, there will always be new ideas and surgical tricks that each of us can incorporate into our own techniques to improve the success for our patients. As with all improvements, you will find that some will work well for you and be absorbed into your own practice, while others may not help as intended.

Learning and growing is part of every practice. The moment that you think you have seen everything is when you will encounter new challenges and unique dilemmas. Every day is another chance to improve and fine-tune your surgical skills, to encounter new challenges, and to provide better care than you did the day before. Almost on a weekly basis, I find that I am still troubled with the frustrations of deciding which technique to perform when indeterminate vasal fluid is encountered. Just when you think that you can accurately predict what you will find, you may discover that your patient who is only 3 years from vasectomy may have thick, toothpaste-like vasal fluid devoid of any sperm and an obvious epididymal blowout, while an older patient, 28 years out, may be found to have whole motile sperm in the vasal fluid on both sides. To make your decision-making even more challenging today, many of our patients will be on testosterone or combinations of herbs and supplements that may be sperm toxic.

I would love to hear what ideas and points you found beneficial to your practice. If you have any thoughts or suggestions, or you have any ideas, tips, or surgical pearls, I encourage you to share them with me to consider for future revisions and to incorporate into my own techniques.

Tucson, AZ, USA   Sheldon H. F. Marks, MD

Acknowledgments

Thank you to all those that have contributed so much over all these decades so that I could have the knowledge and skills to write this book – my professors, colleagues, coworkers, and staff – and especially my family who has tolerated my time away from real life, spending many evenings, weekends, and even holidays typing furiously the many dozens of drafts on my laptop with mountains of photocopied articles piled around the house – Page, Matthew, Jordan, Ally, Caroline, Libby, and my parents Merton and Radee, all of whom, those here and those passed, inspire me every day to be better than I was the day before and to make a difference – the reason I do what I do.

Contents

Chapter 1
Introduction: The Purpose of This Book

There are many excellent reviews and technical guides about vasectomy reversals in journal articles and textbook chapters, yet none go into the step-by-step details, start to finish, of exactly what to do and why to achieve the very best results with a microsurgical vasovasostomy or vasoepididymostomy. Even when I teach courses or write about reversal techniques, time limitations constrict the instructions down to focus on just a few highlights and key points of the microsurgical reversals. This book is written to fill in that void and review my own thought processes and step-by-step surgical techniques, tips, tricks, and pearls that I use every day to perform a vasovasostomy or a vasoepididymostomy. The purpose of this book is not to convince you that a vasectomy reversal is the correct procedure to perform, to highlight the pros and cons of specific controversies, or to provide a detailed history of male reconstructive microsurgery. Likewise, this book does not walk you through the basics of microsurgical skills or techniques. This is a working doctor's hands-on manual based on a career of practical, real-world lessons learned with many thousands of patients over decades. Hopefully, you will learn a number of ideas or points that you will find useful to incorporate into your own reversal techniques to improve your skills, procedures, and knowledge. This book includes the rationale behind my own decision-making as well as how I handle common and uncommon challenges and dilemmas during vasectomy reversals and the care afterward.

Who Am I and Why Am I Qualified to Write This Book About Vasectomy Reversal Techniques?

I was taught many years ago that anytime that you read a book and attend a lecture or a course, your first question should always be "who is this person and why is he qualified so that I should listen to what he has to say?"

© Springer Nature Switzerland AG 2019
S. H. F. Marks, *Vasectomy Reversal*,
https://doi.org/10.1007/978-3-030-00455-2_1

To answer that question, here's a brief summary of who I am. I have performed many thousands of vasectomy reversals going back more than 30 years in my full-time, reversal-only practice. I completed my general surgery at the Mayo Clinic in Rochester, Minnesota, and my urology training at Tufts University/New England Medical Center in Boston more than 3 decades ago. Early in my urology practice, I realized that I was able to achieve a very high success with vasectomy reversals. With that high success and a love of microsurgery, this evolved quickly into my vasectomy reversal practice.

For more than 11 years, I have had the honor of being part of Dr. Peter Schlegel's AUA postgraduate course faculty with Dr. Robert Oates, teaching vasectomy reversal tips and tricks. I have also taught ASRM hands-on microsurgery courses under the leadership of Drs. Mark Sigman and Peter Chan, plus SSMR and ASA talks as well as roundtables on vasovasostomy and vasoepididymostomy techniques. About 15 years ago, I brought into my practice the very talented Dr. Peter Burrows who completed his fellowship with Dr. Lipshultz at Baylor after his residency at the University of Southern California and medical school at Ohio State and the Cleveland Clinic. Together, Peter and I perform reversals on men almost every day from every state in the USA and more than 78 countries around the world.

The Motivation for This Book

This book is a review of my own thought processes and step-by-step techniques, tips, tricks, and pearls when I perform a vasovasostomy or a vasoepididymostomy. As I move further along into the senior years of my practice, I have come to realize that much of what I have learned over all these decades and many thousands of patients will be lost. Several colleagues have encouraged me to share these many tips and ideas from my busy full-time reversal practice to help other doctors who perform reversals. This book provides a means of passing on what I have learned, most often by trial and error or from working and talking with others. My hope is that you will pick and choose what works for you and build on the ideas and advances from this book so that you can improve the care and results for your own reversal patients.

How to Use This Book

If you have performed enough reversals, then I expect that you may not agree with some of the points or ideas in this book. Key surgical principles and patient care apply whatever your technique is. I have come to learn that each expert performs reversals slightly differently, though all are variations on the same themes. For the more experienced urologists, there will be many of the steps that you can skip over, while for others they may find these aspects helpful. I hope that there will be ideas or points that you will find useful and try to incorporate into your own technique. Just the same, you may decide that you don't agree with how I do something or my thoughts or approach, as you have your own technique that works well for you. My intent is to describe what I do and how I handle common and uncommon challenges so that you can consider if any of these are worth trying in your practice. As with any instructions or manual, take what you like and leave the rest. There will be ideas that you may not need today or tomorrow, but someday you might find these pointers helpful to overcome unexpected challenges.

Who is This Book For?

This book is intended for any urologist at any point in their career that is looking to improve their reversal skills, techniques, and knowledge. It's a good idea to always try to be a little bit better today than you were the day before. No matter where you are in your career, it is wise to find out how others do what you do to see if there's any bits of wisdom or insights that you might find useful. My practice has regularly evolved over the years with input and suggestions from others. The moment you think you have it all figured out, your next patient will remind you that as much as you know, there is much that you still have to learn.

What This Book is Not

This book is not a comprehensive, academic treatise on everything reversal. There are plenty of excellent resources that provide a detailed history of microsurgery, how to tie microsutures, or a technical review of intratubular histology in an obstructed epididymis.

Your Suggestions, Corrections, or Tips

I am always excited and eager to improve and learn. If you have any tricks, tips, ideas, or corrections, please contact me directly (shfmarks@gmail.com), so they can be incorporated into any future revisions, courses, or classes and, even more importantly, so that I can modify my own technique to evolve and improve my own patient's care and outcomes.

Thank you to the Leaders

All urologists in the international reversal community should be extremely grateful to those thought leaders who have worked so hard and dedicated themselves to advance the art and science of urologic microsurgery. Some are old, and others are young – a few have left us, while others are still actively contributing to the body of knowledge that we use every day when we perform reversals. From these few – past, present, and future – will come the answers and advances that will allow us to provide even better care for our patients.

As we all know, even an easy reversal is never really easy – it is just easier than the more difficult reversals. To modify the saying of the US Navy SEALs, a good motto for reversal doctors should be "the only easy reversal was yesterday's reversal."

Chapter 2
Who's a Candidate for a Vasectomy Reversal?

The ideal candidate for vasectomy reversal is any relatively healthy male who desires elective reconnection of the vas primarily for the restoration of fertility, most often after prior vasectomy. Vasectomy reversal can also be indicated for iatrogenic damage to the vas, most commonly during inguinal herniorrhaphy, adult or pediatric. If the reversal is for restoration of fertility, then it is important to address with the couple the potential impact of male health, age, lifestyle, and prior fertility as well as the female partner age, health, and fecundity on reversal outcomes. Of course, there are certain medical conditions that would disqualify a patient from having an elective reversal, such as uncorrected high blood pressure, uncontrolled diabetes, or the inability to discontinue anticoagulants. It is important to establish clear and appropriate expectations with the patient and his partner regarding the timeline and outcomes of a vasovasostomy or vasoepididymostomy.

Indications for Vasectomy Reversal

Most vasectomy reversals are performed for the restoration of the patient's fertility post-vasectomy. The majority of patients that we see are with a new female partner following divorce or death of the spouse, while some request a reversal because of a change of heart and desire for more children with the same partner [1, 2]. Specific reasons for wanting the reversal are myriad, anywhere from the usual desire for their own genetic children, after loss of a child, to restoration of their bodily humors or their "chi." There are some men who present with azoospermia which may be a result of intentional or iatrogenic injury of the vas at the time of an inguinal hernia repair, either open or laparoscopically [3]. Other patients may present with idiopathic epididymal obstruction [4].

© Springer Nature Switzerland AG 2019
S. H. F. Marks, *Vasectomy Reversal*,
https://doi.org/10.1007/978-3-030-00455-2_2

The Female Partner

A review of over 3400 patients at our center shows that the average age of the female partner has not increased over decades [5]. Of course, when the reversal is for fertility, it is important to address with the female partner any potential fertility issues such as her age, health, medications, lifestyle, and ovulation status. If there are any questions or concerns or if she is of advanced maternal age, then we usually recommend that she see a reproductive endocrinologist for evaluation to be sure that she is fertile, and a reversal is an appropriate option.

Reversals vs. IVF

Microsurgical vasectomy reversals have fewer risks and are more cost-effective than sperm retrieval with IVF/ICSI for a patient to reestablish his fertility, especially with younger, healthy females with proven prior fertility and no history of any tubal or gynecologic disease that might require assisted reproduction. Plus, there are no added risks to the mother or offspring as a result of the reversal procedure [6–8].

Post–vasectomy Pain Syndrome

A vasectomy reversal can be an effective treatment for selected men with severe, persistent post-vasectomy pain syndrome (PVPS) that is refractory to conservative measures and time. Whether removal of a painful sperm granuloma or treatment of painful, chronic congestive epididymitis via restoration of sperm flow with the repair, most men describe dramatic or total resolution of their post vasectomy pain after a vasectomy reversal. Unlike the other invasive treatments for PVPS, which are destructive in nature, a vasectomy reversal is the only restorative, reconstructive approach [9–13].

References

1. Dickey RM, Pastuszak AW, Hakky TS, Chandrashekar A, Ramasamy R, Lipshultz LI. The evolution of vasectomy reversal. Curr Urol Rep. 2015;16(6):40.
2. Herrel L, Hsiao W. Microsurgical vasovasostomy. Asian J Androl. 2013;15(1):44–8.
3. Schulster ML, Cohn MR, Najari BB, Goldstein M. Microsurgically assisted inguinal hernia repair and simultaneous male fertility procedures: rationale, technique and outcomes. J Urol. 2017;198(5):1168–74.
4. Peng J, Yuan Y, Cui W, Zhang Z, Gao B, Song W, Xin Z. Causes of suspected epididymal obstruction in Chinese men. Urology. 2012;80(6):1258–61.

5. Rehmer JM, Sayles H, Perkins A, Gustin SL, Marks SH, Deibert CM. Female Partner Demographics of Men Seeking Vasectomy Reversal. American Society of Reproductive Medicine Annual Meeting, Salt Lake City, Utah, 2016.
6. Lee R, Li PS, Goldstein M, Tanrikut C, Schattman G, Schlegel PN. A decision analysis of treatments for obstructive azoospermia. Hum Reprod. 2008;23:2043–9.
7. Chan WS, Dixon ME. The "ART" of thromboembolism: a review of assisted reproductive technology and thromboembolic complications. Thromb Res. 2008;121(6):713–26.
8. Huang B, Hu D, Qian K, Ai J, Li Y, Jin L, Zhu G, Zhang H. Is frozen embryo transfer cycle associated with a significantly lower incidence of ectopic pregnancy? An analysis of more than 30,000 cycles. Fertil Steril. 2014;102(5):1345–9.
9. Leslie TA, Illing RO, Cranston DW, et al. The incidence of chronic scrotal pain after vasectomy: a prospective audit. BJU Int. 2007;100:1330–3.
10. Tandon S, Sabanegh E Jr. Chronic pain after vasectomy: a diagnostic and treatment dilemma. BJU Int. 2008;102:166–9.
11. Myers SA, Mershon CE, Fuchs EF. Vasectomy reversal for treatment of the post-vasectomy pain syndrome. J Urol. 1997;157:518–20.
12. Sinha V, Ramasamy R. Post-vasectomy pain syndrome: diagnosis, management and treatment options. Transl Androl Urol. 2017;6(Suppl 1):S44–7.
13. Smith-Harrison LI, Smith RP. Vasectomy reversal for post-vasectomy pain syndrome. Transl Androl Urol. 2017;6(Suppl 1):S10–3.

Chapter 3
Predicting Reversal Success

Predicting success is difficult and cannot be done accurately for an individual preoperatively. Even a good physical exam and detailed history are suggestive at best. Most experts agree that the success of a reversal is primarily dependent on the skill and expertise of the microsurgeon. The highest success rates with patency up to 99.5%, with the fewest complications, are achieved by the most experienced. Another key factor is the accurate intraoperative interpretation of the vasal fluid, both gross and microscopic, which directs whether a vasovasostomy (VV) or vasoepididymostomy (VE) is the correct procedure.

There are many factors that impact on a patient's reversal and subsequent success that includes aspects that the doctor can control and patient-driven variables [1–4]. Of course, knowing about these relevant points allows the surgeon to control and adjust those that are modifiable. Obviously, there are many factors that cannot be controlled or improved upon such as patient age, years since vasectomy, prior fertility or surgeries. This section will address many of these surgeon-related and patient variables that can have potential impact on intraoperative findings and success of the reversal.

Pre-op Counseling

When discussing the patient's potential chances for success, it is important for the surgeon to be honest about their own personal experience, training, and success rates.

When discussing the success of a VV vs. VE, it is important to explain their chances for patency and pregnancy with that patients' obstructive interval and other relevant factors in your own hands [5]. I discuss what I believe to be the pros and cons of my performing their reversal, the option of IVF and quite often offer the names of more local reversal experts that I know and respect.

© Springer Nature Switzerland AG 2019
S. H. F. Marks, *Vasectomy Reversal*,
https://doi.org/10.1007/978-3-030-00455-2_3

Definitions of Success

There is no consistent definition of success in the published literature, which makes comparing techniques and decision-making a challenge. The most appropriate measurement of reversal success is the postoperative return of adequate motile sperm to the ejaculate. The goal of a reversal in our practice is >10 million motile sperm in the ejaculate, though many couples conceive naturally with lower numbers. Many consider 1 million motile sperm a successful reversal [6–8].

Pregnancy is not a good endpoint for measuring success of a vasectomy reversal, even though many patients and even other physicians consider conception a measure of reversal success. Even if the patient has good sperm parameters post-reversal, conception is dependent on many independent female and other male factors beyond the technical success of the reversal. These include female age, health, ovulatory status, weight, male health, medications, testosterone replacement therapy, lifestyle choices, and prior fertility, individually and together, to name a few.

How High Can Reversal Success Be?

In a busy reversal practice, successful return of motile sperm in the ejaculate after a vasovasostomy can be as high as 99.5% and from 70% to 90% for vasoepididymostomy. Of course, statistical success is meaningless to a couple if the reversal doesn't work, and they are the ones with no or inadequate sperm. Just as frustrating for our patients are those with a successful reversal yet are unable to conceive because of other factors. It is important to be honest and up front when talking with patients so that they have reasonable, appropriate expectations regarding patency and pregnancy.

Surgeon Variables

While many of the patient variables cannot be modified, we can control many of the surgeon-related variables. Ideally, the reversal surgeon has done all that can be done to perfect and fine-tune critical microsurgical skills and maximize the facility/equipment and postoperative care aspects of the equation. These are the most important surgeon-based variables.

Microsurgical Skills and Training

Success of any reversal depends on the technical microsurgical skills of the surgeon. As with any challenging surgery, the more experienced the surgeon, the better the outcomes [9–14]. These critical skills should be learned and practiced in the laboratory setting and not on patients who trust us to provide them with the very best care. Training beyond the standard urology residency is essential to offer your patients the very best outcomes by providing important knowledge and skills. These skills are rapidly perishable and so must be maintained in a busy clinical practice or with supplemental laboratory time. Some residency programs provide good hands-on training in microsurgery. Other programs may only perform an infrequent reversal or only allow the doctor to assist and not actually learn and perfect the necessary microsurgical skills.

Time spent learning the subtle nuances of male and female fertility and care before intra-op issues, during, and post-reversal is just as important as knowing how to pass the 70 micron needles or prep the vas for a vasoepididymostomy. Post-residency courses provide the doctor with important skills and knowledge to make those critical pre-op, intra-op, and post-op decisions to ensure the very best outcomes.

Additional training to enhance microsurgical skills can be anything from self-training, a mentorship, an observational experience, a brief refresher course, or a formal 1- to 2-year microsurgical fellowship in male reproductive surgery. Educational and hands-on microsurgical skills and laboratory training, such as the courses offered at ASRM annual conferences or by Dr. Philip Li at Cornell, are a valuable tool for the occasional surgeon who wishes to update his knowledge and improve his skill set [15–18]. A short refresher training course alone does not empower a surgeon with those fine-tuned skills needed to perform a microsurgical vasectomy reversal. Nor does attending a class instantly make you "trained" nor justified to advertise that you are now an expert in microsurgery. This can only be achieved with time and practice.

Microsurgery vs. Macrosurgery

It is generally accepted by male fertility specialists since the 1980s that a microsurgical reversal, though more challenging to learn, perfect, and per-form, will provide a more precise approximation of the layers in a vas-to-vas or vas-to-epididymis anastomosis than a macroscopic repair and so result in a consistently higher success [19–28]. Just because we learned a technique many years before in our residency does not mean that using that technique today is appropriate. Performing vasectomy reversals is not about offering our patients a "good" outcome or doing what's easiest or fastest for the surgeon. We per-form vasectomy reversals to give each and every patient the very best chances for success and so the ability to fulfill their dream to have their own genetic children. As we know, there is nothing more devastating to a couple who wants a child than an unsuccessful reversal. Despite this, there are many urologists that still perform reversals with magnifying loupes and using less successful techniques, all because of a willingness to settle for "good" results. I can't imagine oncologists or cardiac surgeons, or their patients who would be satis-fied with any outcomes less than the very best possible.

Know Your Own Outcomes

If you are performing vasectomy reversals, it is important for you to perform a regular self-audit of your own results, so that you can share these outcomes with your patients considering surgery. It is a disservice to your patients to quote the published success rates of leading reversal experts as if these results were your own. Knowing your own success rates also provides important feedback that you can use to continue successful techniques and decision-making and modify those that are not as successful. We routinely look back at successful and unsuccessful results, focusing on the gross and microscopic fluid findings as well as looking at our technique to try to understand what worked and what didn't and learn how we can improve and be better. Because the success of a reversal can only be determined with many months of monitoring post-reversal semen analyses, this self-audit process can be very time-consuming for the surgeon and the staff and so requires a commitment of resources.

What if I Can Only Perform a Vasovasostomy?

This is a common question by most urologists that perform an occasional reversal. The dilemma is that even with very short obstructive intervals, as soon as 2–3 years post-vasectomy, the need to perform a more challenging VE exists and increases with time. The key is to share these concerns with your prospective patients so that they know and can have reasonable expectations about your own limitations. With an honest, aboveboard approach, surprisingly most patients will choose to have you perform their reversal, well aware of these concerns. In this situation, most reversal experts would agree on two points. First, if you encounter no sperm in the vasal fluid and findings suggestive of epididymal blockage, then you should not try to go ahead and perform a VE if you do not have the experience or skills mastered. It is much more difficult for someone else to perform a VE at a later date if there has been a failed first attempt. Second, we prefer that you try to limit your practice to performing reversals on patients that are just a few years out from vasectomy or those that have sperm granulomas [29].

Experience

As with any technically challenging procedure, the best results will always be with those microsurgeons that have the best experience with thousands of reversals over decades and who continue to perform reversals on a regular basis [9–14]. This allows the doctor to perfect, fine-tune, and maintain those critical skills needed for the very best results. Knowing what to do without the regular, frequent surgical practice allows for these rapidly perishable skills to fade. Long gaps between performing reversals force the doctor to re-perfect those skills on the next patient, which is not in that patient's best interest. The microsurgeon should do whatever is necessary to maintain this skill set. Having years of hands-on experience also provides better judgment with intraoperative decision-making for those patients with indeterminate vasal fluid findings or challenging intraoperative dilemmas or post-vasectomy anatomy.

Specialization

Most vasectomy reversals are performed by general urologists that perform an occasional reversal as part of their busy general urology practice [30]. They have some basic knowledge and limited experience, though they rarely perform enough microsurgery to really perfect and fine-tune their skills. There are some urologists that are fellowship trained but still fall into this category, practicing primarily general urology with an interest in male reproductive medicine and surgery. There are a few urologists that have a full-time, dedicated male reproductive and reversal practice where they perform exclusively vasectomy reversals or where a major part of their practice is reversals. As with any technically challenging skill, the best results with the fewest complications will be seen with those high-volume specialty surgeons who are dedicated to performing the best reversal [8]. Of course, numbers alone are never enough. There are busy reversal doctors that do not perform reversals using state-of-the-art techniques or generally accepted decision-making, such as those that perform only a vasovasostomy on every patient no matter what the vasal fluid shows.

Center/Facility

Ideally, every vasectomy reversal should be performed at the same facility where the critical needs of a reversal are addressed consistently with each and every patient. Though you will always be able to "get by" with a variable surgical assist, lesser or varying equipment or supplies, the best results will usually be seen when you can reliably have access to the same support staff and "tools of the trade" with each and every reversal that you perform.

This includes:

- A top-of-the-line high-powered, XY, double-headed, motorized focus and zoom foot-controlled surgical microscope. The most commonly used leading brands are Leica and Zeiss (Fig. 3.1).
- Properly maintained high-quality microsurgical instruments (Fig. 3.2).
- Specialty microsutures (Fig. 3.3) specifically designed for the unique challenges of microsurgical vasectomy reversals, such as the 10-0 black monofilament nylon double-armed bicurve M.E.T.™ 70 micron needle by Sharpoint ™ (AA-2492).

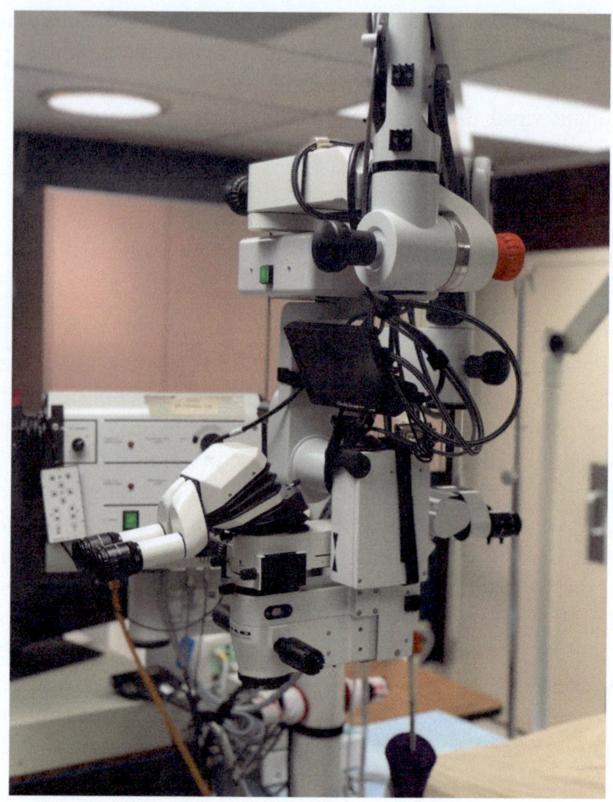

Fig. 3.1 Example of Leica XYdouble-headed, motorized focus and zoom foot-controlled surgical microscope. (Photo Credit: Sheldon Marks)

- A skilled, experienced first assist, ideally the same person from case to case.
- The ability to do whatever needs to be done based on intraoperative findings and challenges, whether a vasovasostomy or vasoepididymostomy, during the reversal without outside pressure or time constraints, whether it will take 2 or 4 h or more.
- An affiliated andrology lab and services, with an experienced and trained andrologist, to assist with real-time microscopic vasal and epididymal fluid analysis, analysis of diagnostic TESE specimens when needed, and sperm cryopreservation when appropriate. The andrologist also plays an important role assisting with interpretation of the post-reversal semen analyses as well as patient education.

In addition, the highest reversal success requires a knowledgeable support staff to assist and participate pre-op and with extended post-reversal patient education and care. Simply performing a reversal and then discharging the patient with minimal post-op guidance and care are not in the patient's best interest.

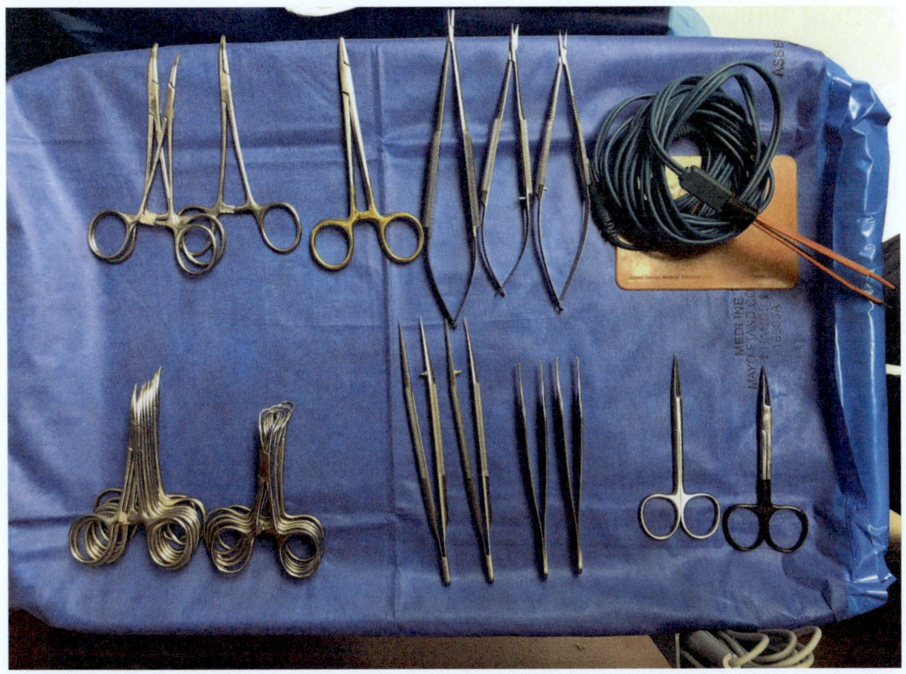

Fig. 3.2 Well-maintained microsurgical instruments. (Photo Credit: Sheldon Marks)

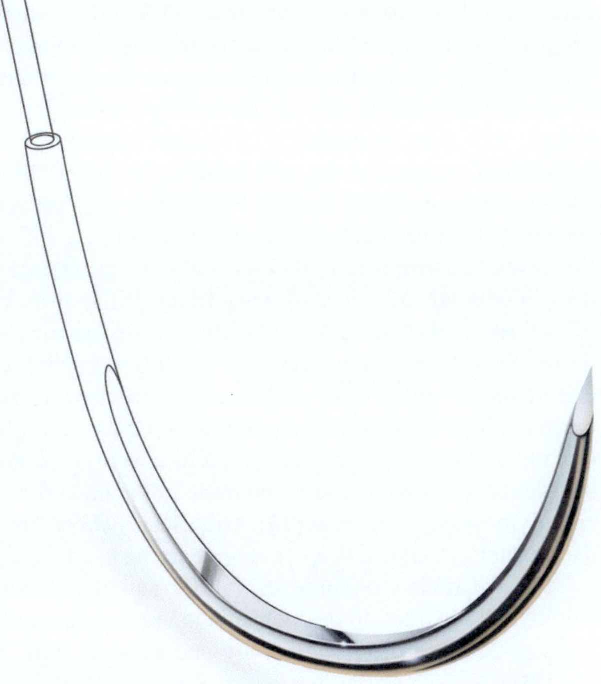

Fig. 3.3 Example of bicurve M.E.T.™ needle by Sharpoint. (Photo Credit: Surgical Specialties Corporation)

Patient Variables and Relevance

There are many patient-driven variables that are out of the surgeon's control that can positively or negatively influence the success of the reversal and whether or not the couple is subsequently able to conceive. Some of these variables can be modified including lifestyle choices, while others such as obstructive interval or age cannot.

Obstructive Interval

A frequent misconception persists that the number of years from vasectomy is the primary variable for predicting success of a vasectomy reversal. There are still surgeons that incorrectly use the obstructive interval as the key determinant to decide on whether to perform a VV or VE. We routinely hear from patients that they were told that the chances for reversal success drop dramatically at 10 years post-vasectomy [31–36]. The post-vasectomy obstructive interval is relevant but not the primary prognostic factor to predict reversal success.

Many doctors frequently quote from the landmark 1991 Vasovasostomy Study Group (VVSG) data, which back in the early 1990s was relevant [37]. However, in more than 25 years since the VVSG data was published, microsurgical reversals have dramatically evolved with improved microsutures, customized microneedles, new and more successful intraoperative decision-making with different thresholds, and surgical techniques for vasovasostomy and vasoepididymostomy, rendering the data from 1976 to 1985 outdated. VVSG data showed that both patency and pregnancy rates after vasovasostomy decrease as the time since vasectomy increases. Progressively decreasing post-reversal patency rates may be a reflection of incorrect vasal fluid assessment and so incorrectly performing a VV when today we would believe that there is evidence of deeper epididymal obstruction, and so a VE is indicated. Likewise, as the technique in the late 1970s for a VE was in its infancy and evolving, it would be safe to say now we are achieving significantly higher success rates than back in the 1970s, as high as 70–90% in experienced hands. Because of this we believe that it is not wise to counsel your patient or make critical decisions based on 30- to 40-year-old data, decision-making, and surgical techniques.

We do know that statistically, the longer the interval since the vasectomy, the more likely the pressure within the epididymal tubules will exceed the capacity of that tubule, resulting in an epididymal blowout with scarring and obstruction and so necessitating a vasoepididymostomy to bypass that blockage. Contemporary data looking at the procedures performed in almost 2700 consecutive patients from our own practice shows a gradual increase in the need for a unilateral or bilateral vaso-epididymostomy (Fig. 3.4) [33]. This clearly shows that at any obstructive interval, there is not a dramatic drop or change in the need for a VV or VE.

A recent review of more than 1200 patients shows that the likelihood of this epididymal obstruction on each side is independent and increases linearly and plateaus at 22 years from vasectomy and beyond (Fig. 3.5) [38]. At an obstructive

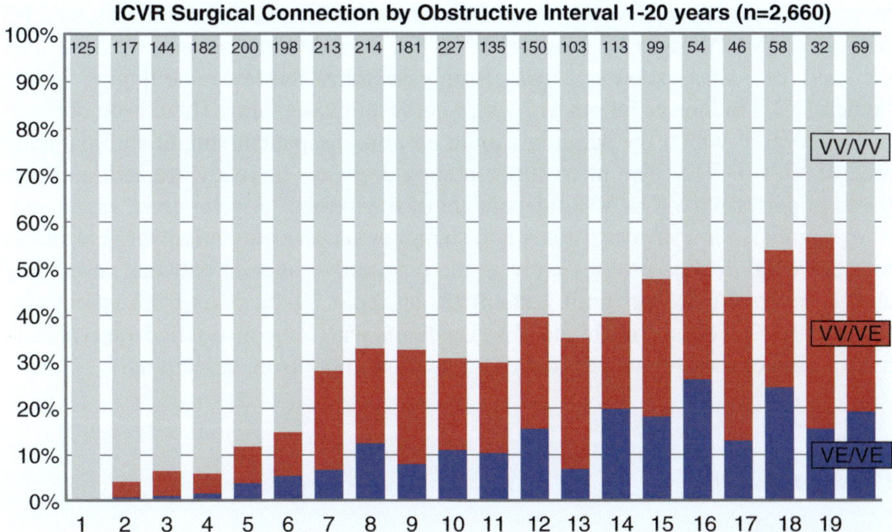

Fig. 3.4 ICVR graph of 2770 patients showing the likelihood of needing a bilateral vasovasostomy, a vasovasostomy/vasoepididymostomy, or a bilateral vasoepididymostomy from 0 to 20 years post-vasectomy

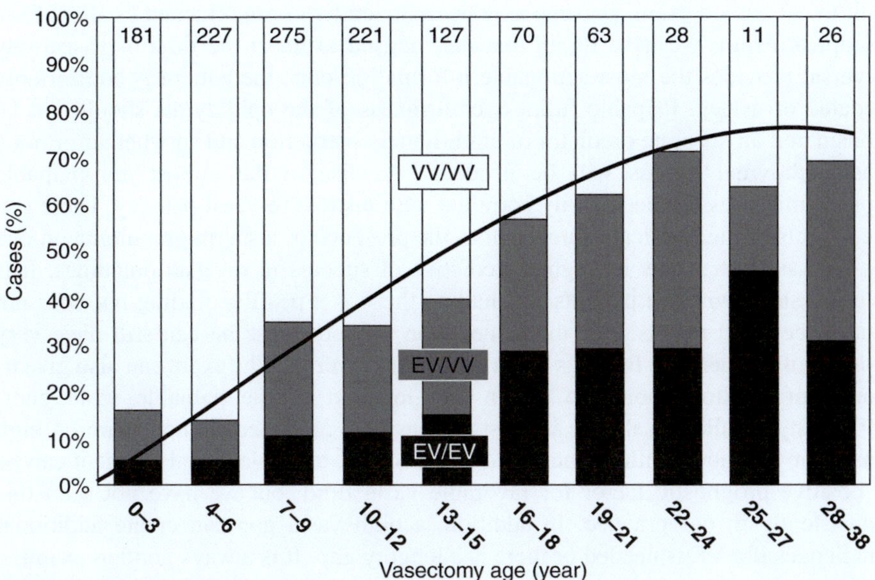

Fig. 3.5 Relationship between vasectomy obstructive interval and type of reversal procedure. The need for vasoepididymostomy (VE) at reversal increases linearly with vasectomy intervals up to 22 years, after which the need for a unilateral or bilateral VE flattens or plateaus

interval of more than 22 years, about 1/3 of men will require bilateral VEs, and 1/3 will need a VV/VE and 1/3 bilateral VVs. For an individual patient, we have seen the need for a VE as soon as 2 years from vasectomy and favorable fluid receiving bilateral VVs in men as far out as 35–42 years from vasectomy. There is no obstructive interval at which the surgeon should assume the patient should automatically receive VVs or VEs. The microsurgeon should always be ready, trained, and prepared to perform a VE or VV independent of the number of years from vasectomy. The prognosis for a vasovasostomy and so higher success after microsurgical vasectomy reversal decline progressively as the obstructive interval between vasectomy and its reversal increases until it stabilizes at about 20–22 years from vasectomy. With 70–90% success for a bilateral VE, patients with long obstructive intervals still have a high chance for success out of 35 years or more from vasectomy.

Physical Exam

The physical exam can be useful to help map the surgical approach and potentially identify any anatomic or postvasectomy findings that may impact on the surgery or outcomes, such as the presence of a sperm granuloma or lengthy vasal gaps. Though it may be helpful and, when possible, encouraged, there are times when the exam in advance may not be possible or may be limited. For some patients, it may be difficult to get a good exam, as some may be quite tender or are reluctant to allow for a complete exam. We have found that the focused exam at the time of vasectomy reversal provides the most actionable information once the patient is comfortably sedated or asleep. Palpable fullness or firmness of the epididymis should not be considered an accurate predictor of epididymal obstruction and so whether or not a vasoepididymal bypass will be needed. Likewise, a flat almost non-palpable epididymis does not necessarily correlate with testicle-to-vasal patency. There can be aspects of the physical exam, such as the presence of a sperm granuloma on one or both sides that may be highly predictive of successful reversal outcomes. It is wise to share with the patients that having these is a positive finding but does not guarantee good results. Just the same, even without these he can still have very positive intraoperative findings and a successful reversal. The exam can also give us some information about the length and location of the palpable vasal gaps. Obviously, smaller vasal gaps are best and easier to reconnect on no tension. A high vasectomy location with an increased length of the testicular vasal segment can be a positive prognostic factor for favorable vasal fluid, but we have not seen this consistently in our practice. In addition, a high vasal gap can create additional challenges if a VE is needed or there is a lengthy gap. It is always good to examine and note the size and consistency of the patient's testicles. Softer, smaller testicles raise concerns over testosterone use or other factors that can compromise sperm production.

Sperm Granulomas

From a reversal point of view, the presence of a sperm granuloma at the vasectomy site is almost always a positive finding. Sperm granulomas are considered to be the "great equalizer" as their presence makes the obstructive interval, even if decades out, irrelevant in most cases [39, 40]. A sperm granuloma is a dense, desmoplastic inflammatory reaction of the body to the post-vasectomy leakage of sperm into the local tissues. The adjacent inflammation often extends out and involves adjacent tissues (Fig. 3.6). Sperm granulomas can be present on one or both sides. These are small to large, from only a few millimeters or several centimeters long. They typically are hard nodules or masses at the vasectomy site. Most of the time, men are not even aware that they have a granuloma or assume it is normal outcome of the vasectomy. Other times, they can be very tender or even quite painful, impacting on normal day-to-day activities, work, or sexual activity.

The fluid that leaks into the tissues would otherwise have built up under a head of pressure and could over time cause an epididymal tubule blowout. This leak of the vasal fluid keeps the testicles and epididymis decompressed at a low-pressure state. Most often, when we transect the testicular vas below the granuloma, we find very favorable vasal fluid independent of the number of years since vasectomy. This fluid is often clear and watery with many sperm. You may encounter the full range from very minimal to copious vasal fluid. Sometimes there are only a rare sperm seen, while other times there may be very high concentrations with very high motility.

The downside to the presence of a sperm granuloma is the concern about the intense inflammatory reaction in and around the granuloma. After the granuloma is excised, we have found that the adjacent inflammation in the granuloma bed can potentially increase the chances for localized vasal inflammation which can present as scarring and possible blockage of the vasal anastomosis. This potential for obstruction is another reason why it is so important to recommend close and regular follow-up semen analyses post-reversal and for the patient to take the post-op anti-inflammation medications, as directed.

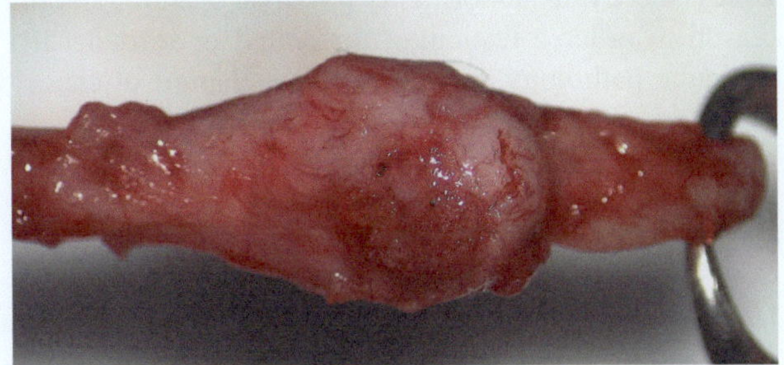

Fig. 3.6 Sperm granuloma and adjacent tissues. (Photo Credit: Sheldon Marks)

Pre-reversal Lab Testing

Most healthy patients do not require any routine pre-reversal laboratory testing. There is no reason to order a shotgun barrage of tests unless there is a specific concern. With a low yield for an otherwise healthy patient, blanket hormone testing is often not covered by insurance and adds an undue financial burden to what, for most, is already significant out-of-pocket expense.

The indication for any pre-reversal testing would be to identify any significant abnormalities or issues that might negatively impact on surgery or fertility outcomes, to postpone the reversal to allow for correction, or to even encourage alternatives to reversal such as sperm retrieval for IVF/ICSI. These are suggested by the patient's past medical or fertility history or physical findings.

Hormone assessment is appropriate if there are concerns over admitted or suspected past or recent testosterone use, to confirm compliance or the effectiveness of corrective HCG or clomiphene therapy pre-reversal. If the patient was unable to father children before vasectomy, then it is recommended to check an FSH. Likewise, if he notes or on examination is found to have small, soft testicle or describes a change in testicle size or consistency, then it makes sense to order hormone levels [41]. Knowing his pre-vasectomy fertility status is very helpful, especially if there were any issues. Many years ago, we performed a reversal on one patient with relatively poor semen parameters post-op. When we notified him of these results, he was actually happy as he told us that these were much better than he had pre-vasectomy.

For the patient that has a large abdomen with significant visceral fat and concerns over an elevated estrogen, then we usually recommend that he check his estradiol and testosterone levels for consideration of possible aromatase inhibitor therapy. There is no reason to test for serum antibodies, as their presence or absence is not helpful for the care and management of the patient.

Role of Testicular Ultrasound or MRI

Unless there is an abnormality found on examination or by patient report, there is no reason to order a testicular ultrasound or scrotal MRI to look for intra- or peri-testicular pathology that might delay, change, or cancel the reversal [42, 43].

Antisperm Antibodies

Discussions regarding antisperm antibodies (ASA) are surrounded by much controversy and misinformation [44–47]. Many experts are unable to agree on the possible impact of ASA on post-reversal fertility. Despite the fact that WHO (fifth edition) notes that up to 50% antibody binding or less is considered normal [44], there are still doctors who incorrectly assume that the simple presence of antisperm antibodies at any level is an abnormal finding and compromises fertility. In our practice, we hear almost weekly from prospective patients who are confused because of comments from other doctors or online forums that "all reversal patients will have ASA, which will prevent the reversal from being successful." When we analyzed ASA and post-reversal fertility data in our practice, we found two key points [45].

1. There was no consistency in patterns or prevalence of ASA after vasectomy reversal. Some men had high levels that stayed high, some had low counts that stayed low, while others had ASA levels that increased, decreased, or fluctuated. The key point is that a single ASA level has no predictive value to future ASA tests with that patient.
2. When considering the clinical relevance of antisperm antibodies, we looked at post-reversal ASA levels and natural conception. We found that there was no significant difference in natural conception and pregnancy rate or time to conception between men with consistently low or no antibodies and those men with consistently high ASA levels. Anecdotally, we had one patient after bilateral VV with documented persistent 100% ASA binding that fathered two children naturally.

There are concerns about ASA's possible negative impact on sperm motility. Typically, the level of ASA binding is not a predictor of whether there are impaired semen parameters such as high agglutination or low progressive motility. So even if a patient is found to have elevated ASA levels (many labs automatically perform ASA testing), the majority will probably have no impact on natural conception following vasectomy reversal. Of course, if you have enough patients, sooner or later you will have the rare patient with significant ASA that impact semen parameters, such as agglutination or unexplained infertility, that would benefit from ART.

Male and Female Variables

Delayed childbearing in today's society is commonplace, which translates to an increasing paternal and maternal age in our patients. In our vasectomy reversal world, we are seeing an increasing number of older men that are remarried and now desire children with their younger wives. Many of the female partners are older after intentionally postponing childbearing for personal reasons, education, or career. In my experience, most couples with one or both older partners are either unaware of the potential consequences of their age on fertility or believe that these concerns will not be relevant to themselves. Advancing maternal age has always been a known issue for conception, carrying to term and the health of the offspring. Recently there has been increased attention given to the role of advanced paternal age and health of the children.

Male Age

More children are being born to older fathers after a vasectomy reversal. It is well known that in general, older men experience a decline in semen analysis parameters relative to their sperm counts at younger ages. Of course, this is statistical probability and may not be relevant to an individual, as we see some men in the 70s with great sperm numbers, while other men in their 40s and 50s can have low sperm counts and motility. It is difficult to assess the true impact of age for an individual as an independent variable without looking at that individuals' trends of their serial parameters over many years pre-reversal. Plus, many older men have confounding factors, independent of age itself but which are associated with increasing age such as a lower testosterone, an elevated estrogen from obesity, various medical and disease states, and reduced sexual function, or are taking various medications that all can impact on spermatogenesis.

There are many studies that suggest that though rare, there are increased risks with increasing paternal age and stillbirth rates, birth defects such as cleft palate, some malignancies, neurodevelopmental disorders, and schizophrenia in their offspring [48–50]. Of course, these risks are minor relative to female age-related issues. Though these risks from advanced paternal age are reported, we have not seen this in our busy practice with thousands of post-reversal children. We have to admit we are not systematically following up to assess these specific problems as we rely on voluntary patient reporting of pregnancy, children, and any health issues or problems with the offspring.

Female Age and Health

The impact of female age on fertility is well documented as an important predictor of pregnancy. The best rates for post-reversal conception and delivery are with healthy females under the age of 35. Spousal age is important for men with an obstructive interval of more than 15 years. The lowest pregnancy rates will be seen with an older, nulliparous female partner [51–55]. Unless you are performing the reversal exclusively for management of PVPS, it is important to obtain a medical and fertility history of the female partner during the pre-reversal assessment. This should include female age, any prior or current health concerns, previous fecundity, or issues with ovulation that can impact on the likelihood for natural conception after reversal. We share with prospective patients how her age and these concerns can negatively impact on whether or not she can become pregnant or carry to term, with a higher rate of miscarriage and birth defects in older women, even if the reversal is a success with good sperm counts and motility. Our reproductive endocrinology colleagues will confirm that this is real but caution that these concerns vary widely from person to person. In our practice, if the female partner is of advanced maternal age or has any menstrual or fertility issues, we encourage them to see a reproductive endocrinologist for a pre-reversal assessment.

Prior Male and Female Fecundity

It has been clearly established, and common sense would support that nulliparous women will have lower success conceiving after successful vasectomy reversal than those women with proven prior conception and childbearing. The same increased rates of successful fertility will be seen by men who have prior proven ability to father children. The very best chances for conception after reversal are with couples where the females have proven successful fertility with the same male partner as compared to a woman with a new partner [56, 57].

BMI/Obesity

There is a general consensus that there is a negative relationship between body mass index (BMI) and lowered semen parameters as a result of endocrine dysregulation, increased scrotal temperature from increased scrotal fat, and a more sedentary lifestyle [58–66]. We looked at BMI in our own practice and potential impact on intraoperative vasal fluid and post-reversal sperm parameters and found that BMI does not predict for intraoperative vasal fluid findings or post-reversal outcomes [62]. We do try to obtain testosterone and estradiol levels for men with significantly elevated BMI from increased abdominal girth, with the recommendation that if the estradiol is considerably elevated, then discuss the initiation of an aromatase inhibitor to block the conversion of testosterone to estradiol. This should boost sperm production and allow for a more rapid weight loss with an appropriate regimen of diet and exercise over time.

Anyone who has performed enough reversals knows that the technical aspects of a microsurgical reversal can be far more challenging and usually more time-consuming with patients who have a significantly elevated BMI. Some of these mechanical difficulties we encounter that can impact on vasectomy reversal include:

- The increased size of the patient can change the angle of approach, from an ideal horizontal surgical plane to having to operate at a 30- to 45-degree angle.
- Because of the patient's added girth, depending on the focal distance and surgical microscope lenses used, there are times when you may have to elevate the microscope to its maximum height and, if you are sitting, look up into the oculars throughout the case or have to stand when you would normally sit to perform the reversal.
- Many men with increased BMI have sleep apnea or disordered breathing which can introduce significant "body breathing" and so added scrotal movement with associated challenges during the reversal.

Lifestyle

There are countless ways that a patient's lifestyle can negatively impact on their sperm quality and fertility and so their perceived success of the reversal. Even when these are pointed out with concerns and consequences, many patients either refuse to change or are unable to alter these sperm-compromising habits [67–69].

Alcohol

Alcohol in moderation is thought not to be an issue for most men. However, excessive drinking raises concerns over multi-organ toxicity and a negative impact on sperm parameters and DNA integrity from compromised spermatogenesis. We tell patients to limit their alcohol intake to no more than two drinks a night and avoid binge drinking. Many that have a drinking problem will not likely admit their addiction or will refuse to change [70].

Marijuana

We have seen an increase with the use of marijuana in our reversal patients, as many states now have legalized medical marijuana or even recreational use marijuana.

When talking with our patients, we discuss that daily or regular marijuana use lowers sperm counts and can damage the DNA as compared to occasional or nonusers [71, 72]. When this has been pointed out to patients who are regular users from those states where medical or recreational marijuana is legal, the men and their wives almost universally are surprised. The classic response was "well how can it be bad for me if it is legal?" Another concern (and opportunity for education) was when one reversal patient told me, "so I understand that it is not good for me but it's okay of my wife to smoke daily, right?"

Tobacco

Tobacco in all forms is associated with a negative impact on semen parameters, fertility, a compromise of sperm DNA, and issues with wound healing [73]. We looked at patency and pregnancy rates of almost 2000 of our reversal patients that smoked compared to nonsmoking reversal patients. We found, to our surprise, no increased risks for post-op anastomotic scarring, although we did note a lower conception rate in partners of smokers with comparable sperm parameters to our matched nonsmokers [74].

Relevant Past and Current Medical History

Most serious and chronic health issues have the potential to compromise sperm production, function, and fertility by the nature of the disease itself and from the medications to treat the illness. Some of the most common medical problems that can impact fertility include diabetes, hypertension, obesity, and associated metabolic disorders as well as rheumatoid arthritis and other autoimmune diseases.

The list of commonly used medications, prescription and over-the-counter, as well as supplements that are hormonally active and sperm toxic or disrupt male reproduction increases daily and is beyond the intent of this book. Just as dangerous are medications and supplements that can increase risks for intraoperative and post-reversal bleeding, interfere with the medications given at the time of the reversal, or compromise wound healing. Many patients do not consider herbal supplements or vitamins to be relevant and so do not share that they are taking these, even when asked.

Of course, cancer and any associated surgery, radiation, and chemotherapy can all have a well-known temporary or permanently negative impact on fertility. With dramatic improvement in survival, the impact on future fertility from gonadotoxic treatments has become even more relevant [75].

Testosterone Replacement Therapy

Most reversal experts have had a dramatic increase in the number of reversal patients that are currently on or have recently been taking testosterone replacement therapy. Its seems that testosterone therapy is almost an epidemic, no longer limited to older men but now including young healthy men. It is not uncommon to have patients who are firefighters, police, or even those with sedentary jobs whose doctors thought they would be better on testosterone. And then there are so many longevity and men's health centers that seem willing to start almost any man on testosterone. When we discuss the concerns about testosterone and the impact on fertility and the reversal, most men are surprised, unaware of this consequence. When we become aware of current or past use, we explain our concerns and how their testosterone use can impact on intraoperative decision-making, outcomes, and possible banking. We also use that opportunity to work with and educate their prescribing doctors who are most often open and receptive to this new information. There have been a few doctors over the years that have told me that I am wrong and that there is no evidence or literature to support the fact that testosterone therapy can negatively impact on sperm production.

Testosterone and Intra-op Decision-Making

As we all know, testosterone replacement therapy can severely and sometimes completely suppress sperm production [76–78]. This makes intraoperative interpretation of the vasal fluid difficult as we are left to guess if the absence of sperm is because of suppression from the testosterone or because of deeper epididymal obstruction. Of course, each patient is different, and, in your practice, you will find men who have been on testosterone for many years with good counts of whole, motile sperm in the vasal fluid at the time of their reversal. Other times, you will encounter men who have been on testosterone for a short time and have total suppression.

To Stop or Not to Stop?

The majority of men are willing to stop the testosterone replacement before their reversal and start clomiphene and/or HCG (human chorionic gonadotropin), though there are always a few that will insist on staying on the testosterone, aware of the concerns and issues. Most are honest and open about the use of testosterone, though on occasion we will discover a patient that still denies he is taking testosterone even when his sperm production is severely suppressed and with labs that confirm exogenous testosterone. The longer the duration on testosterone, the longer it will take to rebound and recover, with or without HCG.

Patient Honesty and TRT

With testosterone clinics openly advertising testosterone use as part of our society's regular conversation, the use of testosterone is more commonplace and accepted. Even with that, there are still some men who are covertly using testosterone, whether legally prescribed from a physician or bought illegally through a gym or other sources. As with all patient care, you can only work with the information you are given. Even in the face of irrefutable results with a testosterone of >1800 and a suppressed FSH and LH, some men will still deny they are on testosterone.

Impact of Vasectomy Technique and Complications on Reversibility

An overly aggressive vasectomy with excision or damage to an excessive length of the vas is the most common technique that makes a vasectomy reversal more challenging. Most often, at the time of a reversal, we encounter a 1 or 2 cm segment of the vas that was excised or damaged by cautery, clips, or ties from the vasectomy. There are occasions when we see up to 5–6 cm or more of the vas that has been excised or damaged, making the reversal even more challenging as we try to free up enough length to be able to perform the anastomosis on no tension. This becomes even more problematic when a vasoepididymostomy is needed, and the end of the abdominal vas is located high in the scrotum. On occasion we will find a small segment excised but with metal clips across the vas several centimeters above and below the damage, forcing us to excise and perform the anastomosis across the lengthy gap.

Hematoma

The damage from post-vasectomy bleeding and hematoma formation around the vas and in the scrotum can lead to dense peri-vasal scarring that can make reversal more challenging and time-consuming. The blood causes damage as it dissects through tissues as well as from inflammation and scarring from the desmoplastic reaction and reabsorption that can increase risks for ischemic consequences to the vas and repair. The average incidence for bleeding occurs in about less than 1–2% of vasectomies [79].

Infection

Just as with bleeding, infection in the spermatic cord or scrotum after a vasectomy can cause significant peri-vasal and peri-testicular scarring with obliteration of normal tissue planes. This damage can be localized to small section of the cord or be a lengthy process along the entire spermatic cord and around the testicle/epididymis on that side. The post-infection scarring can dramatically increase the difficulty of performing a reversal as well as post-reversal complications. Infections after vasectomy are very uncommon with an incidence of 1–2% [79].

Lengthy Vasectomy Gap

The presence of an excessive length of damaged vas or lengthy gaps between the abdominal and testicular vas from an aggressive vasectomy can make reversal surgery especially challenging, as the surgeon has to work to perform a tension-free anastomosis without permanently elevating the testicle high up in the scrotum.

Low Vasectomy Site

There are times when you will discover that the vasectomy was performed very low down in the deep convoluted vas. This creates unique challenges as you work to create a good anastomosis between a very small, often eccentric lumen with minimal surrounding vasal muscularis and no adventitia to the straight abdominal vas with a thick muscularis (Fig. 3.7). This almost feels at times like a routine end-to-side vasoepididymostomy. It is reasonable to transect every few millimeters as needed in the apex of the arch or mid loop to try and identify a central lumen.

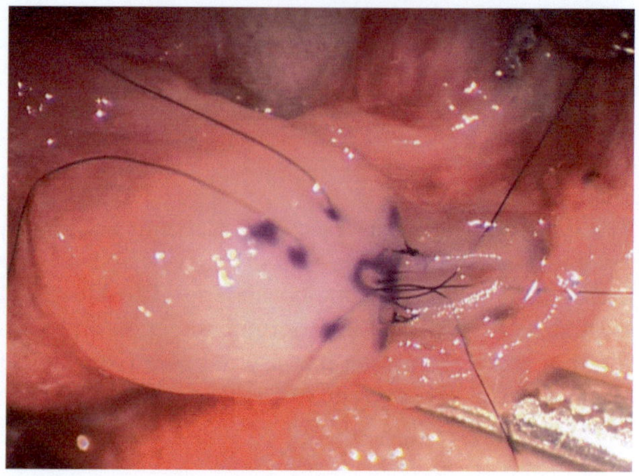

Fig. 3.7 Very low vasectomyinto the deep convoluted vas. Note minimal muscularis on the testicular vas. (Photo Credit: Sheldon Marks)

Post–vasectomy Pain

Persistent pain (post vasectomy pain syndrome (PVPS)) is one of the most frustrating and misunderstood post-vasectomy complications. Patients often present with severe testicular or epididymal pain associated with a broad constellation of symptoms. These can sometimes include pain before, during, or after ejaculation; pain with sitting or exercise and extreme, debilitating tenderness; and pain with pressure or movement, often not localized to a specific point. Performing a reversal for pain or for fertility with pain requires additional attention to address the probable etiology whether obstructive epididymitis, sperm granuloma, or other issues. These patients also can involve significantly increased interactions with your staff before and after their reversal [80–86].

Repeat Second Vasectomy

There are instances when a second vasectomy is performed for the reappearance of sperm in the ejaculate post vasectomy from spontaneous recanalization or persistent sperm after a technically flawed first vasectomy. A reversal after a "double vasectomy" is rarely routine. On occasion, some doctors simply re-resect a small vasal segment of the vas adjacent to the prior vasectomy, and so the reversal is not significantly more difficult. More commonly, the doctor will resect lengthy segments of the vas, aggressively cauterize long portions of the vas and distal vasal lumens, or place multiple ties or metal clips high up and low on the vas, with the intent to prevent spontaneous reconnection. This obviously creates significant challenges to performing the anastomosis on no tension.

Even more difficult, there are doctors that perform a second vasectomy by resecting a vasal segment at a separate location along the vas, which can be near or sometimes quite a distance from the earlier vasectomy site. This creates the concerns about having to perform two reversals on each vas with concerns over the possibility of a compromised blood supply to the middle vasal segment (Fig. 3.8). The other solution is to resect the entire middle segment between the two vasectomy sites, then bringing together the abdominal vas from the upper vasectomy to the testicular vas of the lower vasectomy. This then introduces the issue of having to perform the reversal across a lengthy vasal gap. It is never a favorable prognostic

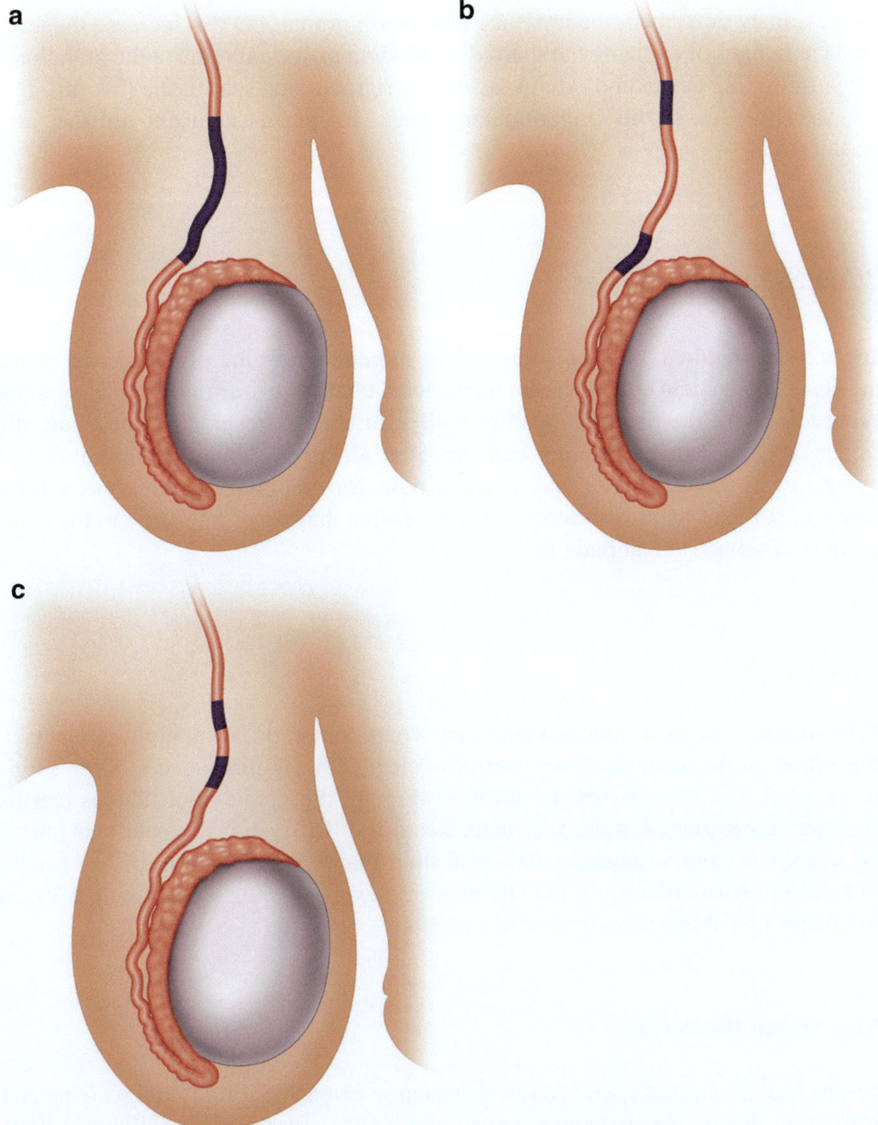

Fig. 3.8 Three scenarios seen with a repeat vasectomy. (**a**) Lengthy vasal gap. (**b**) Vasectomy sites far apart. (**c**) Adjacent vasectomy sites

sign when the patient tells you that the vasectomy doctor proudly announced that he was going to remove or damage a lengthy segment of vas to be sure that "this does not happen again."

Sperm Granuloma

As previously described, the presence of a sperm granuloma can increase the technical challenges of excising the scarred vasal segment as you remove the granuloma and surrounding dense and often vascular peri-granuloma scar tissue [39, 40]. It is not wise to leave this inflammatory mass in place, adjacent to the new anastomosis.

Other Scrotal Surgeries

Any scrotal, inguinal, or even some pelvic surgeries have the potential to damage the vas or the testicle and so create unexpected challenges for the reversal surgeon trying to restore the patient's fertility with a vasectomy reversal. In addition, the surgery and subsequent healing can make an already challenging microsurgical reversal even more difficult and increase risks for complications. This is a brief review of some of the more common surgeries that may be of relevance to the management of your reversal patient.

Spermatocele

Previous excision of a spermatocele can wreak havoc on an attempted reversal. Depending on the location of the spermatocele and the aggressiveness of the surgical excision, the flow of sperm and fluid through the epididymal tubules can be restricted or obstructed at the spermatocelectomy site. Even if the patient is only a few years out from vasectomy, the vasal fluid may show no sperm or parts, with evidence of obstruction up to the spermatocele excision site, necessitating a VE in the tubules just above this surgical obstruction.

Prior Sperm Retrieval

Pre-reversal attempts at sperm retrieval can cause extensive epididymal scarring and obstruction, depending on the specific technique, and so force a vasoepididymostomy. Just as challenging, the reversal surgeon may encounter dense peri-testicular or epididymal scarring or damage, often with a loss of normal tissue planes from the prior sperm retrieval attempt. You may have patients with multiple sperm retrievals before they come for reversal. Many times, scarring from prior sperm retrieval can slow down the reversal as you have to dissect delicately through the dense scar to identify an underlying tubule for the VE, often above the epididymal injury.

Hydrocele

Prior hydrocele surgery or even past aspiration with sclerotherapy can result in dramatic and significant thickening and scarring of the tunica vaginalis with dense peri-testicular and peri-epididymal scarring. If the patient requires a VE on that side, the surgeon may have difficulties just delivering the testicle and then freeing up the underlying epididymis from the overlying scar. Often after hydrocele surgery, you may find that the tunica vaginalis is partially or totally absent or can be densely adherent to the underlying tunica albuginea with obliteration of the tunical space. This can make dissection out of the epididymis and identification of underlying tubules especially challenging and time-consuming. Even if the tunica vaginalis is not scarred to the tunica albuginea, one might encounter a very thickened and scarred tunica vaginalis.

Varicocele

Varicocele ligation surgery, whether subinguinal, inguinal, retroperitoneal, or laparoscopic, rarely interferes with the vasectomy reversal itself. There are concerns that an aggressive varicocelectomy might potentially compromise the peri-vasal and testicular blood flow with an unintended or intentional division of the testicular artery, relying on collateral arterial vessels to provide blood supply to the testis. This can result in a more tenuous testicular blood supply and increase the risks for ischemic changes post-reversal. There are also situations with an inguinal varicocele repair where the abdominal vas can be inadvertently damaged or fixed within the inguinal scar. This can be a challenge if the vasectomy was performed high or with a lengthy vasal gap and is especially a problem if a VE is indicated on that side.

Orchiopexy for Undescended Testicle or Torsion

Prior orchiopexy for treatment of an undescended testicle or for management and prevention of testicular torsion can impact on a vasectomy reversal in two ways. First, the corrective surgery can significantly increase peri-vasal and peri-testicular scarring. When we explore the hemiscrotum at the time of reversal, we commonly encounter a loss of normal tissue planes in men with this prior surgery, making the surgery even more challenging. If the orchiopexy was performed as infant, the patient may not even be aware of the procedure. The second impact of this surgery at the time of the reversal relates to the markedly reduced spermatogenesis with incomplete maturation we can find in the undescended testicle. This can make intra-op decision-making confusing when trying to decide if the absence of sperm in the vasal fluid is from epididymal obstruction or from nonproduction of sperm.

References

1. Nagler HM, Jung H. Factors predicting successful microsurgical vasectomy reversal. Urol Clin North Am. 2009;36(3):383–90.
2. Bolduc S, Fischer MA, Deceuninck G, Thabet M. Factors predicting overall success: a review of 747 microsurgical vasovasostomies. Can Urol Assoc J. 2007;1(4):388–94.
3. Elzanaty S, Dohle GR. Vasovasostomy and predictors of vasal patency: a systematic review. Scand J Urol Nephrol. 2012;46(4):241–6.
4. Shin YS, Kim SD, Park JK. Preoperative factors influencing postoperative results after vasovasostomy. World J Mens Health. 2012;30(3):177–82.
5. Kovac JR, Lipshultz LI. Factors to consider for informed consent prior to vasectomy reversal. Asian J Androl. 2016;18(3):372.
6. Crosnoe LE, Kim ED, Perkins AR, Marks MB, Burrows PJ, Marks SH. Angled vas cutter for vasovasostomy: technique and results. Fertil Steril. 2014;101(3):636–9.
7. Perkins A, Marks M, Burrows P, Marks S. Sperm kinetics following vasectomy reversal. Androl. 2012;33(Suppl2):42.
8. Silber SJ, Grotjan HE. Microscopic vasectomy reversal 30 years later: a summary of 4010 cases by the same surgeon. J Androl. 2004;25(6):845–59.
9. Aikoye A, Harilingam M, Khushal A. The impact of high surgical volume on outcomes from laparoscopic (totally extra peritoneal) inguinal hernia repair. J Clin Diagn Res. 2015;9(6):PC15–6.
10. Anderson BR, Ciarleglio AJ, Cohen DJ, Lai WW, Neidell M, Hall M, Glied SA, Bacha EA. The Norwood operation: relative effects of surgeon and institutional volume on outcomes and resource utilization. Cardiol Young. 2015;14:1–10.
11. David EA, Cooke DT, Chen Y, Perry A, Canter RJ, Cress R. Surgery in high-volume hospitals not commission on cancer accreditation leads to increased cancer-specific survival for early-stage lung cancer. Am J Surg. 2015;210(4):643–7.
12. Esquivel MM, Molina G, Uribe-Leitz T, Lipsitz SR, Rose J, Bickler SW, Gawande AA, Haynes AB, Weiser TG. Proposed minimum rates of surgery to support desirable health outcomes: an observational study based on four strategies. Lancet. 2015;385(Suppl2):S12.
13. Kalakoti P, Missios S, Menger R, Kukreja S, Konar S, Nanda A. Association of risk factors with unfavorable outcomes after resection of adult benign intradural spine tumors and the effect of hospital volume on outcomes: an analysis of 18,297 patients across 774 US hospitals using the National Inpatient Sample (2002-2011). Neurosurg Focus. 2015;39(2):E4.
14. Shuhaiber J, Isaacs AJ, Sedrakyan A. The effect of center volume on in-hospital mortality after aortic and mitral valve surgical procedures: a population-based study. Ann Thorac Surg. 2015;100(4):1340–6.
15. Mehta A, Li PS. Male infertility microsurgical training. Asian J Androl. 2013;15(1):61–6.
16. Scallon SE, Fairholm DJ, Cochrane DD, Taylor DC. Evaluation of the operating room as a surgical teaching venue. Can J Surg. 1992;35(2):173–6.
17. Grober ED, Hamstra SJ, Wanzel KR, Reznick RK, Matsumoto ED, et al. Laboratory based training in urological microsurgery with bench model simulators: a randomized controlled trial evaluating the durability of technical skill. J Urol. 2004;172:378–81.
18. Li PS, Ramasamy R, Goldstein M. Male Infertility Microsurgical Training. In: Sandlow JI, editor. Microsurgery for Fertility Specialists. New York: Springer; 2012.

19. Dickey RM, Pastuszak AW, Hakky TS, Chandrashekar A, Ramasamy R, Lipshultz LI. The evolution of vasectomy reversal. Curr Urol Rep. 2015;16(6):40.
20. Baker K, Sabaneugh E Jr. Obstructive azoospermia: reconstructive techniques and results. Clinics. 2013;68(Suppl1):61–73.
21. Dewire DM, Lawson RK. Experience with macroscopic vasectomy reversal at the medical college of Wisconsin. Wis Med J. 1994;93(3):107–9.
22. Feber KM, Ruiz HE. Vasovasostomy: macroscopic approach and retrospective review. Tech Urol. 1999;5(1):8–11.
23. Fox M. Vasectomy reversal—microsurgery for best results. Br J Urol. 1994;73(4):449–53.
24. Gopi SS, Townell NH. Vasectomy reversal: is the microscope really essential? Scott Med J. 2007;52(2):18–20.
25. Herrel LA, Goodman M, Goldstein M, Hsiao W. Outcomes of microsurgical vasovasostomy for vasectomy reversal: a meta-analysis and systematic review. Urology. 2015;85(4):819–25.
26. Jee SH, Hong YK. One-layer vasovasostomy: microsurgical versus loupe-assisted. Fertil Steril. 2010;94(6):2308–11.
27. Safarinejad MR, Lashkari MH, Asgari SA, Farshi A, Babaei AR. Comparison of macroscopic one-layer over number 1 nylon suture vasovasostomy with the standard two- layer microsurgical procedure. Hum Fertil (Camb). 2013;16(3):194–9.
28. Schwarzer JU. Vasectomy reversal using a microsurgical three-layer technique: one surgeon's experience over 18 years with 1300 patients. Int J Androl. 2012;35(5):706–13.
29. Chawla A, O'Brien J, Lisi M, Zini A, Jarvi K. Should all urologist performing vasectomy reversal be able to perform vasoepididymostomies if required? J Urol. 2004;172(3):1048–50.
30. Crain DS, Roberts JL, Amling CL. Practice patterns in vasectomy reversal surgery: results of a questionnaire study among practicing urologist. J Urol. 2004;171(1):311–5.
31. Kolettis PN, Sabanegh ES, D'amico AM, Box L, Sebesta M, Burns JR. Outcomes for vasectomy reversal performed after obstructive intervals of at least 10 years. Urology. 2002;60(5):885–8.
32. Matthews GJ, Schlegel PN, Goldstein M. Patency following microsurgical vasoepididymostomy and vasovasostomy: temporal considerations. J Urol. 1995;154(6):2070–3.
33. Marks SHF, Burrows PJ, Cropp AR, Ax RL, McCauley TC. Obstructive interval should not be a deterrent in vasectomy reversal. Androl. 2008;(Suppl):21.
34. Peng J, Zhang Z, Yuan Y, Cui W, Song W. Pregnancy and live birth rates after microsurgical vasoepididymostomy for azoospermic patients with epididymal obstruction. Hum Reprod. 2017;32(2):284–9.
35. Harza M, Voinea S, Ismail G, Gagiu C, Baston C, Preda A, Manea I, Priporeanu T, Sinescu I. Predictive factors for natural pregnancy after microsurgical reconstruction in patients with primary epididymal obstructive azoospermia. Int J Endocrinol. 2014;2014:873527.
36. Peng J, Yuan Y, Zhang Z, Cui W, Song W, Gao B. Microsurgical vasoepididymostomy is an effective treatment for azoospermic patients with epididymal obstruction and prior failure to achieve pregnancy by sperm retrieval with intracytoplasmic sperm injection. Hum Reprod. 2014;29(1):1–7.
37. Belker AM, Thomas AJ Jr, Fuchs EF, Konnak JW, Sharlip ID. Results of 1,469 microsurgical vasectomy reversals by the Vasovasostomy Study Group. J Urol. 1991;145(3):505–11.
38. Mui P, Perkins A, Burrows PJ, Marks SF, Turek PJ. The need for epididymostomy at vasectomy reversal plateaus in older vasectomies: a study of 1229 cases. Androl. 2014;2(1):25–9.
39. Boorjian S, Lipkin M, Goldstein M. The impact of obstructive interval and sperm granuloma on outcome of vasectomy reversal. J Urol. 2004;171(1):304–6.
40. Maghelia A, Rais-Bahrami S, Kempkensteffen C, Weiske WH, Miller K, Hinz S. Impact of obstructive interval and sperm granuloma on patency and pregnancy after vasectomy reversal. Int J Androl. 2010;33(5):730–5.
41. Hsiao W, Sultan R, Lee R, Goldstein M. Increased follicle-stimulating hormone is associated with higher assisted reproduction use after vasectomy reversal. J Urol. 2011;185(6):2266–71.
42. Donkol RH. Imaging in male-factor obstructive infertility. World J Radiol. 2010;2(5):172–9.

43. Ammar T, Sidhu PS, Wilkins CJ. Male infertility: the role of imaging in diagnosis and management. Br J Radiol. 2012;85(Spec Iss 1):S59–68.
44. World Health Organization. WHO laboratory manual for the examination and processing of human semn. 5th ed. Geneva: WHO Press; 2010.
45. Marks M, Perkins A, Russell H, Burrows P, Marks S. Antisperm antibodies: prevalence, patterns and impact on natural conception following vasectomy reversal. Fertil Steril. 2013;100(3):S375.
46. Carbone DJ Jr, Shah A, Thomas AJ Jr, Agarwal A. Partial obstruction, not antisperm antibodies, causing infertility after vasovasostomy. J Urol. 1998;159(3):827–30.
47. Newton RA. IgG antisperm antibodies attached to sperm do not correlate with infertility following vasovasostomy. Microsurgery. 1998;9(4):278–80.
48. Sharma R, Agarwal A, Rohra VK, Assidi M, Abu-Elmagd M, Turki RF. Effects of increased paternal age on sperm quality, reproductive outcome and associated epigenetic risks to offspring. Reprod Biol Endocrinol. 2015;13:35.
49. Almeida S, Rato L, Sousa M, Alves MG, Oliveira PF. Fertility and Sperm Quality in the Aging Male. Curr Pharm Des. 2017;23(30):4429–37.
50. Sigman M. Introduction: What to do with older prospective fathers: the risks of advanced paternal age. Fertil Steril. 2017;107(2):299–300.
51. Deck AJ, Berger RE. Should vasectomy reversal be performed in men with older female partners? J Urol. 2000;163(1):105–6.
52. Gerrard ER Jr, Sandlow JI, Oster RA, Burns JR, Box LC, Koettis PN. Effect of female partner age on pregnancy rates after vasectomy reversal. Fertil Steril. 2007;87(6):1340–4.
53. Hinz S, Rais-Bahrami S, Kempkensteffen C, Weiske WH, Schrader M, Magheli A. Fertility rates following vasectomy reversal: importance of age of the female partner. Urol Int. 2008;81(4):416–20.
54. Kolettis PN, Sebanegh ES, Nalesnik JG, D'Amico AM, Box LC, Burns JR. Pregnancy outcomes after vasectomy reversal for female partners 35 years old or older. J Urol. 2003;169(6):2250–2.
55. Hsieh MH, Meng MV, Turek PJ. Markov modeling of vasectomy reversal and ART for infertility: how do obstructive interval and female partner age influence cost effectiveness? Fertil Steril. 2007;88(4):840–6.
56. Chan PT, Goldstein M. Superior outcomes of microsurgical vasectomy reversal in men with the same female partners. Fertil Steril. 2004;81(5):1371–4.
57. Ostrowski KA, Polackwich AS, Kent J, Conlin MJ, Hedges JC, Fuchs EF. Higher outcomes of vasectomy reversal in men with the same female partner as before vasectomy. J Urol. 2015;193(1):245–7.
58. Eisenberg ML, Kim S, Chen Z, Sundaram R, Schisterman EF, Buck Louis GM. The relationship between male BMI and waist circumference on sperm quality data from the LIFE study. Hum Reprod. 2014;29(2):193–200.
59. Hinz S, Rais-Bahrami S, Kempkensteffen C, Weiske WH, Miller K, Magheli A. Effect of obesity on sex hormone levels, antisperm antibodies, and fertility after vasectomy reversal. Urology. 2010;76(4):851–6.
60. Jensen TK, Andersson AM, Jorgensen N, Andersen AG, Carlsen E, Petersen JH, Skakkebaek NE. Body mass index in relation to semen quality and reproductive hormones among 1558 Danish men. Fertil Steril. 2004;82(4):863–70.
61. Macdonald AA, Stewart AW, Farquhar CM. Body mass index in relation to semen quality and reproductive hormones in New Zealand men: a cross sectional study in fertility clinics. Hum Reprod. 2013;28(12):3178–87.
62. Marks M, Perkins A, Burrows P, Marks S. Body mass index does not predict for intraoperative findings or post-operative outcomes with vasectomy reversal. Androl. 2012;33(Suppl2):35.
63. Kato JM, Iuamoto LR, Suguita FY, Essu FF, Andraus W. Impact of Obesity and Surgical Skills in Laparoscopic Totally Extraperitoneal Hernioplasty. Arq Bras Cir Dig. 2017;30(3):169–72.
64. Amri R, Bordeianou LG, Sylla P, Berger DL. Obesity, outcomes and quality of care: body mass index increases the risk of wound-related complications in colon cancer surgery. Am J Surg. 2014;207(1):17–23.

65. Srinivasan D, La Marca F, Than KD, Patel RD, Park P. Perioperative characteristics and complications in obese patients undergoing anterior cervical fusion surgery. J Clin Neurosci. 2014;21(7):1159–62.
66. McPherson NO, Lane M. Male obesity and subfertility, is it really about increased adiposity? Asian J Androl. 2015;17(3):450–8.
67. Rossi BV, Abusief M, Missmer SA. Modifiable risk factors and infertility: what are the connections? Am J Lifestyle Med. 2014;10(4):220–31.
68. Sharma R, Biedenharn KR, Fedor JM, Argawal A. Lifestyle factors and reproductive health: taking control of your fertility. Reprod Biol Endocrinol. 2013;11:66.
69. Pacey AA, Povey AC, Clyma JA, McNamee R, Moore HD, Baillie H, Cherry NM. Participating Centres of Chaps-UK. Modifiable and non-modifiable risk factors for poor sperm morphology. Hum Reprod. 2014;29(8):1629–36.
70. Jensen TK, Gottscchau M, Madsen JO, Andersson AM, Lassen TH, Skakkebaek NE, Swan SH, Priskorn L, Juul A, Jorgensen N. Habitual alcohol consumption associated with reduced semen quality and changes in reproductive hormones; a cross-sectional study among 1221 young Danish men. BMJ Open. 2014;4(9):e005462.
71. Gundersen TD, Jorgensen N, Andersson AM, Bang AK, Nordkap L, Skakkebaek NE, Priskorn L, Juul A, Jensen TK. Association between use of marijuana and male reproductive hormones and semen quality: a study among 1215 healthy young men. Am J Epidemiol. 2015;182(6):473–81.
72. Eisenberg ML. Invited Commentary: The Association between Marijuana Use and Male Reproductive Health 2015. Am J Epidemiol. 2015;182(6):482–4.
73. van Dongen J, Tekle FB, van Roijen JH. Pregnancy rate after vasectomy reversal in a contemporary series: influence of smoking, semen quality and post-surgical use of assisted reproductive techniques. BJU Int. 2012;110(4):562–7.
74. Perkins, AR, Burrows PJ, McCauley TC, Ax RL and Marks SF. Smoking decreases pregnancy rates of vasectomy reversal patients. 64th Ann. Mtng Amer Soc Reprod Med. 2008. Abstract.
75. Agarwal A, Said TM. Implications of systemic malignancies on human fertility. Reprod Biomed Online. 2004;9(6):673–9.
76. Kovac JR, Scovell J, Ramasamy R, Rajanahally S, Coward RM, Smith RP, Lipshultz LI. Men regret anabolic steroid use due to lack of comprehension regarding the consequences on future fertility. Andrologia. 2015;47(8):872–8.
77. Kovac JR, Lipshultz LI. Basic concepts and recent advancements in the study of male fertility. Asian J Androl. 2016;18(3):331.
78. Coward RM, Mata DA, Smith RP, Kovac JR, Lipshultz LI. Vasectomy reversal outcomes in men previously on testosterone supplementation therapy. Urology. 2014;84(6):1335–40.
79. Johnson D, Sandlow JI. Vasectomy: tips and tricks. Transl Androl Urol. 2017;6(4):704–9.
80. Leslie TA, Illing RO, Cranston DW, et al. The incidence of chronic scrotal pain after vasectomy: a prospective audit. BJU Int. 2007;100:1330–3.
81. Tandon S, Sabanegh E Jr. Chronic pain after vasectomy: a diagnostic and treatment dilemma. BJU Int. 2008;102:166–9.
82. Myers SA, Mershon CE, Fuchs EF. Vasectomy reversal for treatment of the post-vasectomy pain syndrome. J Urol. 1997;157:518–20.
83. Lee JY, Cho KS, Lee SH, Cho HJ, Cho JM, Oh CY, Han JH, Lee KS, Kim TH, Lee SW. A comparison of epididymectomy with vasectomy reversal for the surgical treatment of postvasectomy pain syndrome. Int Urol Nephrol. 2014;46(3):531–7.
84. Lee JY, Chang JS, Lee SH, Ham WS, Cho HJ, Yoo TK, Lee KS, Kim TH, Moon HS, Choi HY, Lee SW. Efficacy of vasectomy reversal according to patency for the surgical treatment of postvasectomy pain syndrome. Int J Impot Res. 2012;24(5):202–5.
85. Sinha V, Ramasamy R. Post-vasectomy pain syndrome: diagnosis, management and treatment options. Transl Androl Urol. 2017;6(Suppl 1):S44–7.
86. Smith-Harrison LI, Smith RP. Vasectomy reversal for post-vasectomy pain syndrome. Transl Androl Urol. 2017;6(Suppl 1):S10–3.

Chapter 4
Pre-reversal Preparations

Making the effort to plan and prepare before the reversal can reduce potential risks and complications as well as improve patient care and reversal outcomes. Obtaining proper consent for the reversal is important to address standard as well as reversal-related risks. Discussing the consents with the patient and partner should be face-to-face by the surgeon and not delegated to ancillary, facility, or other staff. This is an excellent time to help build a rapport with the patient and establish reasonable expectations. Providing the patient with verbal and written pre-reversal instructions, especially regarding medications, supplements, and blood thinners, increases the chances of compliance and reduces the likelihood for complications. It is important to be sure that the patient is medically cleared for the surgery, with discussions with his doctors if appropriate. In addition, taking the time to arrange for appropriate operating room time, preprepared surgery packs, the correct microsutures, instruments, OR table, and chairs well as a consistent surgical team ensures an easier reversal experience for both the surgeon and patient while providing better results. The most commonly used types of anesthesia by top experts are general anesthesia or mild conscious sedation with local anesthesia. All together, these presurgical preparations maximize the reversal outcomes which is the ultimate goal of the surgery.

Consenting the Reversal

When consenting for the vasectomy reversal, face-to-face discussion with your patient is important. Do not delegate this critical task to ancillary, facility, support staff, or nurses. The key is to manage the patient and his partner's expectations with information and build a rapport, so they have realistic expectations about the reversal, follow-up, fertility, and pregnancy. The consent can actually be useful as a tool to help the patient understand potential risks and complications, so that they can become a more informed member of the "team." [1] We have found that many men express that they do not want to read or discuss the worst-case scenarios as they

© Springer Nature Switzerland AG 2019

S. H. F. Marks, *Vasectomy Reversal*,

https://doi.org/10.1007/978-3-030-00455-2_4

find it upsetting to even think or talk about these issues, and so we make it a standard policy to offer a copy of the consents to all patients.

Of course, in addition to the standard surgical and medication/anesthetic risks, you should review reversal-specific risks and complications, which may require additional surgeries or procedures. These risks, similar to those after a vasectomy, include the possible failure of the repair, scarring, pain, injury, atrophy or loss of one or both testicles, hydrocele, bleeding, and infection [2–4]. When talking about the benefits, alternatives such as sperm retrieval with IVF/ICSI, risks, and potential complications of the surgery, the surgeon should emphasize that there are no guarantees with the outcomes of the reversal and that though most risks are rare, they can be serious and have life-long consequences such as post-vasectomy reversal pain [5] or testicular atrophy. It is important to review that the goal of the reversal is restoration of sperm flow back into the ejaculate and that there are a multitude of other male factors and sperm production issues that can influence outcomes. Just as important, it is wise to note that a well-performed reversal with successful results still does not guarantee pregnancy or a healthy baby.

Pre-reversal Instructions and Care

To maximize your surgical results and minimize risks for infection and bleeding, it is important that you provide critical pre-reversal instructions to your patient. The goal is to minimize any modifiable risks and potential complications. Of course, compliance is always an issue, so we provide written, emailed, and then a verbal review of all pre-reversal instructions and guidelines [6, 7]. These preoperative guidelines include standard instructions before any procedure or surgery as well as vasectomy reversal specific.

This is also a good time to review important post-reversal restrictions and precautions so that they don't plan a weekend horseback riding event or triathlon for a few days after the surgery. Despite this written and verbal review, there are occasions when men will still have taken aspirin for several days leading up to the surgery or started multiple herbal supplements to "help with healing or fertility." If the patient has any significant medical or cardiac history, it is best to coordinate and receive clearance in advance from the patient's doctors before the reversal. If there are any concerns or questions, then it may be best to talk directly with the patient's physician. Many doctors do not understand the nature of a vasectomy reversal and incorrectly assume it is either similar to a quick vasectomy or that it is a major surgery. This is a brief list of the general instructions that we review with our patients preoperatively.

Medications and Supplements

It is emphasized to all patients that they are not allowed to take any medications that can inhibit platelets or compromise bleeding starting 10 days before the reversal. This includes prescription, over-the-counter, vitamins, and supplements. Obviously, this includes all aspirin-containing medications, most NSAIDs, blood thinners, as well as "natural" supplements to include fish oil, high-dose garlic, parsley, and wheat grass extract. If the patient is on aspirin or other blood thinners for a medical reason, prescribed by their doctor, then we ask their doctor for medical or cardiac clearance to stop these pre- and post-reversal to minimize intraoperative and postsurgical risks for bleeding.

If they need to be on an NSAID for a musculoskeletal injury or chronic pain, then we recommend that they can take either celecoxib or meloxicam as neither compromises platelet function [8].

If the patient takes any vitamins or supplements, we ask them to stop them all 10 days before the surgery as well to be sure that there are no potential interactions with prescribed medications and sedatives or any unknown side effects from the ingredients.

Our nurses then review every medication that the patient takes routinely, so we can instruct them which they should continue and which medications to hold, when to stop and restart after the reversal. We ask the patient to not start any new medications, vitamins, or supplements before surgery without checking with our office first, to be sure that they do not begin anything that will potentially increase risks for the surgery or compromise the sperm findings [9].

It is essential that you review again preoperatively at the time of surgery what medications or supplements they are taking as many times men will be on a medication that they did not report or may have started new medications since they completed the preoperative medical history. It is not wise to assume that they are still taking only what they told you 3–6 weeks ago, as it often changes. Many men, in anticipation of the reversal will start new supplements or herbs thinking that this will boost fertility or healing. Surprisingly, many patients are started on a variety of supplements by their well-meaning primary care doctors, naturopaths, or integrative doctors who think that they are helping improve healing and the outcomes. Many couples are encouraged to take special fertility products by well-meaning friends and family. Unfortunately, quite often these can compromise platelet function, serve as a blood thinner or can negatively impact on sperm quality.

General Preparation

If the patient has any significant past or current medical or cardiac history, it is best to coordinate and receive clearance in advance from the patient's doctors before the reversal. If there are any concerns or questions, then it may be best to talk directly with the patient's physician. We have found over the years that most doctors do not understand the nature of a vasectomy reversal and incorrectly assume it is either similar to a quick vasectomy or that it is a major surgery. A phone call provides an opportunity to educate that physician as well as ensure the best care for your patient.

We ask the patients not to self-shave their scrotum for several days pre-reversal, as we will take care of the shaving and prep at the time of surgery. If they have any metal genital piercings we ask that they remove them or replace them with plastic ones until after the surgery.

We request that the patients wear comfortable, loose pants and bring an athletic supporter or compression shorts to wear over their underwear as a way of providing compression, to minimize movement and to hold the ice bags not directly against the scrotal skin. Because they will be applying ice bags under the supporter and over their underwear, we have found it is best for the patient to wear boxer briefs rather than briefs as they expose the thigh skin directly to the ice bags.

The office provides additional guidance on lifestyle activities to avoid, which can compromise sperm quality such as excessive heat [10]. We also provide written sperm banking information with a review of the various options and scenarios to consider for further discussion before the reversal.

We ask that our patients remain NPO (nulla per os) for several hours pre-reversal. For early AM cases, we ask that they remain NPO after midnight with minimal clear liquids up until 2–3 h before the reversal, and for the PM case, the patient can eat or drink up to 5 AM. Most urologists will have to work with the established guidelines at their own institution or center. We have found that it has not been problem for our patients to skip their breakfast before surgery.

In the pre-reversal discussion and after the physician's review and signing of the consents, the patient is given an oral celecoxib 200 mg or meloxicam 15 mg to prevent excess post-reversal inflammation and reduce any discomfort with 30 cc of water and an oral low-dose diazepam to provide some relaxation.

Scheduling OR Time

This topic is relevant for vasectomy reversals that are performed in a hospital or surgery center where your reversal will be one of many cases in a busy OR schedule with other surgeons, before and to follow your surgery. Because of this it is important for the surgeon to block out enough OR time so that the correct procedure, with whatever challenges are encountered, can be performed even if it takes longer than anticipated or scheduled without pressure to move fast from other surgeons or facility administrators. As we all know, a significant delay with an earlier surgery can wreak havoc on a tightly scheduled busy OR day if there are multiple cases to follow. Each reversal surgeon should be able to estimate approximately how long a standard, uneventful reversal will take. At our center, most reversals take on average from 2 to 2.5 h. There are times, however, such as with complicated VEs, redo reversals, the presence of large, dense granulomas, significant scarring, or other anatomic challenges, that can unexpectedly add an hour or two to the anticipated operative time.

Surgery Packs

We have found that it is very helpful and reduces costs considerably to use a premade custom vasectomy reversal pack for every case. We have developed our own content list over several decades to include what we need for our reversals.

Table 4.1 Content list of our premade vasectomy reversal surgical packs

Blade No. 15
Bowl 16 oz.
Bowl 32 oz.
Bowl 8 oz. (#2)
Cover mayo stand, 23 × 54
Eye spears, package of 10
Gauze 4 × 4, (#40 total)
Surgical gown
IV cath 24G × ¾ inch (#2)
Labels
Needle 27gG
Pediatric drape
Ruler
Skin marker
Syringe 10ML
Syringe 10ML control top
Syringe 3 ml (#2)
Table cover 44 × 76
OR towels (#8)
Vented bag

The content list of our sterilized pack is shown in Table 4.1. Of course, each surgeon can and should customize the contents of their own surgery pack to suit their own specific needs. It is wise to have your surgery team pay close attention to the items included in the premade packs over time to be sure they are maintaining consistency and quality. We discover on a regular basis, without notice, that some of the contents in the pack, such as the gauze 4 × 4's or the skin markers, will be changed to a lesser quality product or some items may no longer be included.

OR Monitors for Staff Observation

We have two TV monitors in the operating suite connected through a high-definition video camera attached to the surgical optics which allows the nurses, support staff, or observers to view the reversal and see what the surgeon sees real-time. This allows the nurses to be aware of what we are doing so they can be proactive with whatever sutures, instruments, or andrology services will be required. In addition, in our surgical suite, we have the ability to view whatever the andrologist is seeing on the laboratory microscope. With this, the surgeon can see the andrologist's view of the vasal fluid looking for sperm or parts to better decide whether to perform a vasovasostomy or vasoepididymostomy. This is especially helpful in situations when there are indeterminate microscopic findings of the vasal fluid. Having the laboratory microscopic viewing in the OR is also helpful when training others about decision-making based on the analysis of the vasal fluid.

Surgical Table and Chairs

OR Table

The operating table must be a stable, consistent platform that allows for the surgeon and assistant to sit or stand comfortably, with the ability to easily access the bipolar foot pedal as well as the surgical microscope focus, zoom, and XY movement foot pedals. Most standard OR tables are not usable, especially for those surgeons that sit during the reversal as the central table pedestal blocks the ability of the surgeon and assistant to sit with their legs and feet positioned under the patient. If you are using different facilities or OR rooms from case to case, it is important that the surgeon check out any OR table they plan to use before the reversal begins to be sure that the OR table fits their specific needs. Some surgeons have built their own tables, while others modify existing tables with foot extensions.

Surgical Chairs

The surgeon and assistant's OR chair is critical to provide comfortable seating throughout a multi-hour procedure. The correct chair will allow for easy access to foot pedals as well as forearm support throughout the reversal. The specifics of the OR chair are very personal to the surgeon's height, weight, and preferences. You should try out many before deciding on what OR chair works best for you.

Surgical Team: First Assist and Circulator

In an ideal world, it is always best to have the same first assistant/surgical tech with every reversal so that they learn and know your needs and routines. This will allow you both to move smoothly through the reversal without any delays as the experienced assistant will proactively know what to anticipate and be prepared, always one step ahead. In our experience, a consistent and knowledgeable assist will reduce operative time and improve the technical reversal. Try to avoid the default of using whomever is assigned to assist you that day or a less experienced colleague.

Patient Positioning

The goal is to keep the patient safe and secure in a comfortable, supine position with his head, neck, and arms supported with clean, dry padding. It is important to be sure that there is no excessive stretching of the arms to protect the brachial plexus or compression on any potential pressure points, especially the neck, shoulders, elbows, hips, and knees. For most patients we prefer to tuck, support, and secure both arms, though on occasions for large men, we may use arm boards. For large barrel-chested men, we have found that sometimes when they are lying flat on their back on the OR table, their shoulders are often elevated off the support of the padding on the table, leading to shoulder or back discomfort or even pain. Preemptively placing padded supports under their shoulders will help reduce or eliminate this pain for large or overweight patients.

Prep and Drape

The location of the prep and positioning of the drapes are important in case you need to extend the incision or make additional high scrotal or inguinal incisions. Even for routine reversals, we usually extend the area of the prep to include the inguinal regions for those rare instances when a more proximal exploration, extension of the incision, or additional incisions may be needed.

Anesthesia Options

The most common anesthesia choices for a vasectomy reversal are general anesthesia or conscious IV sedation with a local anesthetic block. The goal of any anesthesia approach is to keep the patient safe, comfortable, pain-free and provide a steady surgical platform. Surgeon preference usually dictates the anesthesia technique. Other factors that dictate the specific anesthesia for a patient include patient request, medical issues that may limit anesthetic options, or reversal-specific issues. For example, general anesthesia may be more appropriate if you anticipate a more challenging case, as can be expected with prior scrotal trauma and surgeries or with a challenging redo "salvage" reversal. With increasing concerns over cost control, there is more interest to consider less expensive options, though I would caution that this may be reasonable only for selected and highly motivated patients with appropriate safety considerations.

General Anesthesia

General anesthesia allows the surgeon to move a bit faster with the patient asleep. It also provides for a better surgical environment for teaching. The concerns with general anesthesia are the rare but serous risks, the potential for incomplete local blocks, and the increased costs for the anesthesiologist, anesthesia equipment, and medications as well as post-anesthesia nausea/vomiting, which is obviously not desirable in a fresh post-reversal patient.

Mild Conscious Sedation

If you opt for mild conscious IV sedation, which is my preferred technique, most doctors use low-dose, intermittent IV fentanyl and versed, with the patient continuously monitored, with supplemental local tissue and cord blocks. I have found this technique to be very effective and well tolerated by the patients with minimal risks and an easy recovery.

Oral Meds Alone

There are some doctors that preoperatively give the patient a handful of multiple oral medications alone and then supplement with additional oral meds as needed throughout the case. There are obviously concerns about this because of variable absorption and effectiveness, especially if any additional issues or challenges are encountered during the reversal.

Local Anesthetic to Supplement or as the Sole Anesthetic

It is wise to use local anesthetic before surgery and as needed throughout the reversal to block any pain and keep the patient comfortable during and after the surgery. There has been some recent attention to the use of local as the only anesthetic modality with good results [11]. I have used this "local-only" technique on a few patients over the years who have either requested this approach or had medical issues where sedation or general anesthesia was contraindicated. However, these patients were heavily screened and quite motivated. For most of my patients, I have been happy that I was not using local alone and instead was using mild IV sedation or general anesthesia.

Tools

Having the right tools for the job makes for an easier procedure with better success and fewer problems or complications. As with techniques, over time each surgeon will discover what microinstruments, microsutures, and optics work best. Talking with other experts and spending time watching them perform reversals will often provide information about tools and products that they use that you may want to try. Over many years, I have not been impressed with new vendors offering what they claim to be the same quality at a fraction of the price of what we routinely use.

Microinstruments

It is smart to always use the best quality, task-specific microinstruments. In our experience the lesser quality, cheap instruments are cheap for a reason and should be avoided. We have found these discount instruments to be less precise, often fail and break easily – usually at the worst possible time during your reversal. When selecting microinstruments, it is more important to consider the purchase as an investment in the outcomes of your surgery and not a cost. These low-cost instruments may be cheap initially but when they fail, or you have to replace them frequently, then it becomes clear why it is wise to purchase high-quality microinstruments up-front from a reputable dealer. See *Appendix 1* for a master list with photos of our trays with all the microinstruments that we use for vasovasostomy and vasoepididymostomy. Some quality providers have pre-packaged microsurgical trays specific to vasovasostomy and vasoepididymostomy which include most of the microinstruments that you will need.

Surgical Field Drapes

We have found that using the standard blue background drapes can add time-consuming challenges when you need to hunt for missing microneedles after they accidentally pop off the suture or simply migrate. Instead, we use a modified white eye drape, white towels and drapes and the white instrument wipe technique for vasal fixation. We have found that the use of these white drapes for the background makes it much easier and faster to locate the microneedle that inadvertently pops off and "disappears" or the errant wandering suture, saving time and the added expense of having to open a new suture packet.

Micropens

The biggest challenge when placing the microdots is to find a consistently high-quality microtipped surgical pen. Over the years we have encountered frequent problems with inconsistency in the pen tips, even with the same brand from the same manufacturer within the same lot or box. Despite many micropens being labeled as "micro," most are not. For a number of years, we found a simple fine-tipped pen to be the best microtip, that is, until there was a change in factories and the same model pen was no longer microtipped. We currently use a fine-tipped Devon Skin Marker (KS 77642412) though there are times when the microdot looks more like a paw print than a dot. We also use a blunt-tipped skin marker to highlight the arch of the epididymal tubule when performing VEs, to better define and visualize the open edge of the tubule.

Fig. 4.1 Foam from the suture packets with dots placed to secure the microneedles after use and throughout the reversal for the needle count at the completion of the surgery. (Photo Credit: Sheldon Marks)

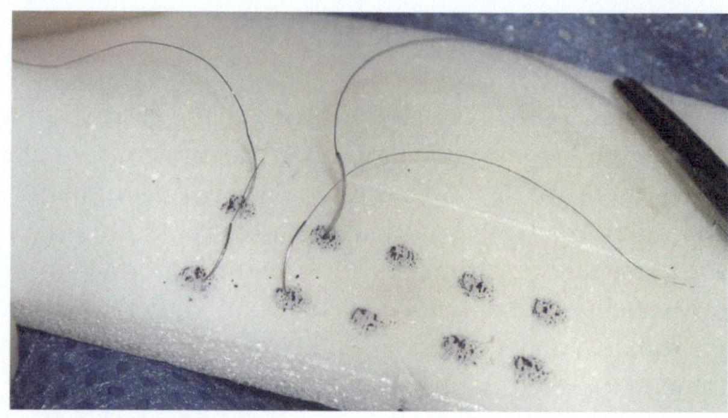

Foam to Secure the Used Microneedles

We have found it very helpful during and at the end of the reversal to place all microneedles as they are being used or when done onto the foam that holds the microneedles within each suture packet (Fig. 4.1). We place two rows of microdots with the finer-tipped marker down one side for the used microneedles and then another two separate dots to secure and hold the 9–0 and 7–0 needles after being used on the first side, before they are needed on the other side. This dramatically reduces the chances of losing any of the microneedles before the final needle count at the end of the case and also keeps the 9–0 and 7–0 needles sharp and accessible when needed for the second anastomosis.

Needles and Sutures

In an ideal world, you should be able to choose the specific microsutures which are so critical to the success of your reversals. However, with so many large institutions locked into national buying groups, many times your options and choices may be restricted. Whenever possible you should do all that you can to be able to obtain the ideal microsutures needed to perform a VV or VE. It is never wise to settle for adequate when you can use the best.

Microneedles

Top experts use task-specific needles to allow for precise placement of the sutures with the least trauma to surrounding tissues. The challenge is to use the finest needle possible to pass the suture through specific tissues. If the needle is too delicate, then it can easily bend, or the tip will quickly become dull. If the needle is too thick and rigid, then the needle will cause more trauma and damage to tissues. For the mucosal layer, we use 70-micron needles, and for the muscularis, we use 100-micron needles. The specific needle tips are critical in microsurgical reversals, as the

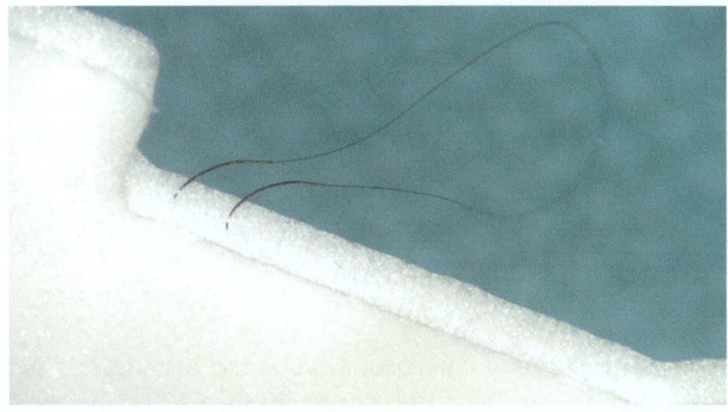

Fig. 4.2 Specialty microsutures specifically designed for the unique challenges of microsurgical vasectomy reversals, such as the 10–0 black monofilament nylon double-armed bicurve M.E.T. 70-micron needle by Sharpoint (AA-2492). (Photo Credit: Sheldon Marks)

standard taper point is not sharp enough to pass easily through the muscularis and a cutting needle is too traumatic for the tissues. Specialty microneedles specially engineered for the unique challenges of vasectomy reversals are the best and most commonly used by top experts. The most commonly used needle for vasectomy reversals is the bicurve needle (95°/107°) with the M.E.T. ™ needle tip from Sharpoint (Fig. 4.2). This task-specific needle is an angled combination of a cutting and taper tip that allows for easy penetration though the mucosa and the muscularis with minimal tissue damage. The bicurve angle allows for a more natural passage of the needle out through the mucosa when performing a VV or VE. The muscularis uses a ½ circle cutting needle.

Microsutures

The goal is to use the smallest diameter nonabsorbable monofilament suture you can without compromising the repair. Nylon (polyamide polymer) is the most commonly used suture material for the microsurgical approximation of the vasal and epididymal tissues with a VV or VE. Nonabsorbable sutures are preferred as their presence in the tissues minimizes inflammation. Monofilament products allow for less resistance when being passed through tissues with lower risks for infection. We use the finest suture we can that will achieve the goal to reduce the amount of foreign body reaction and tissue trauma. For the mucosal layer, we use a 10–0 nylon, for the muscularis a 9–0 nylon, and for the adventitia a 7–0 nylon suture.

Surgical Microscope

The higher-quality surgical microscopes, such as those by Leica or Zeiss, use the best glass optics and so provide clearer visualization under high power with less eye strain. The double-headed adjustable eyepieces are ideal and allow for 180° visualization by your assistant. XY foot control of zoom and focus improves efficiency and allows for real-time adjustments as needed during the surgery. Some of the newer surgical microscopes use very strong lights which are hotter and so dry out the tissue more quickly. Most often you will have to use the surgical microscope in your facility. If you have the option to buy a surgical microscope, it is wise to try out several models from different manufacturers to find the one that best fits your needs.

Laboratory Microscope

As with a surgical microscope, choose the highest quality laboratory microscope that you can get. Whether for use in the OR or in your lab, the quality of the optics is best when you choose a laboratory microscope from a well-known vendor with an established reputation for quality and service. The laboratory microscope we use is a Nikon binocular light microscope, phase-contrast substage condenser with 10 × oculars and 40 × planar adjusted, and 100 × oil immersion objective lenses.

Hemostasis

It is important to maintain good hemostasis real-time throughout the reversal as even minimally bleeding vessels can distort the tissues and cause blood to track up along the vas and create a cord hematoma. This can be very painful postoperatively and potentially lead to increased scarring and inflammation. It is best to control any bleeding real-time as the reversal proceeds and not wait until the end, as it is usually much more challenging to find small blood vessels later on that are the source of any bleeding within a clot or bloody tissues. I am always on the lookout throughout the reversal for new bleeding and reexamine each side again several times before closing. On occasion, you may discover a small artery or vein that was not seen earlier or that was not bleeding when you last checked.

Cautery and Bipolar

The general rule with cautery and bipolar is to always use the lowest possible settings for the shortest duration that will allow for the effective control of the bleeding. We prefer a microneedle tip for the cautery. For microvessel bleeding, it is best to use microbipolar forceps to more precisely control any bleeding near or on the vas. Do not use cautery near the vas or epididymis. Instead, use short pulses of the bipolar. When performing a vasoepididymostomy, we reduce the bipolar level down to the lowest level that is effective. Do not use bipolar directly on the transected face of the vas, the lumen mucosa, or the opened epididymal tubule as this can cause unnecessary injury to the tissues. Excessive cautery will cause tissue damage and

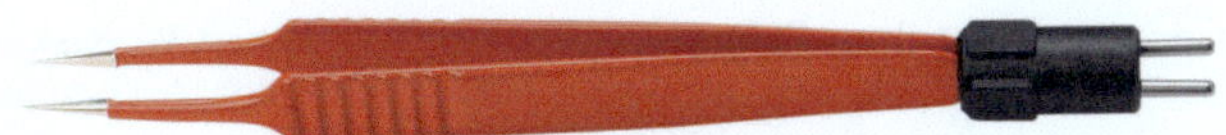

Fig. 4.3 Our preferred bipolar tominimize charring and provide more accurate delivery of energy to control bleeding – a straight pointed tip, 0.25 mm tip diameter jeweler's bipolar forceps, nonstick Noble metal, straight pointed tip, 0.25 mm tip diameter. (Photo Credit: Accurate Surgical and Scientific Instruments, Corp. [ASSI])

can compromise the reversal by causing increased inflammation and tissue ischemia. Because charred blood and tissue frequently accumulates on the tips of the bipolar or cautery, reducing effectiveness, it is important to keep an eye on these tips and regularly clean them to remove any charred tissue. The microtip cautery can be purchased with a Teflon tip. I prefer the special Noble metal bipolar (ASSI. BPNS11223) which minimizes charred accumulation, allowing for control of the bleeding at a lower energy level (Fig. 4.3). These Noble tipped bipolar forceps are fine-tipped but are not available in a true microtip size for bipolar.

Irrigation to Prevent Desiccation

Frequent irrigation of the repair is essential to keep the exposed vas and tissues moist and from drying out and so becoming desiccated under the high-power microscope lights and low humidity in the operating room environment. We use regular pulses of heparinized saline or LR by the assistant via a 24-gauge Angiocath. It is important as well to irrigate with a small pulse of fluid just as you tie down the first knot of every stitch to wash any clots or debris and allow for a clean, direct coaptation of the tissues.

References

1. Kovac JR, Lipshultz LI. Factors to consider for informed consent prior to vasectomy reversal. Asian J Androl. 2016;18(3):372.
2. Lowe G. Optimizing outcomes in vasectomy: how to ensure sterility and prevent complications. Transl Androl Urol. 2016;5(2):176–80.
3. Awsare NS, Krishnan J, Boustead GB, Hanbury DC, McNicholas TA. Complications of vasectomy. Ann R Coll Surg Engl. 2005;87:406–10.
4. Adams CE, Wald M. Risks and complications of vasectomy. Urol Clin North Am. 2009;36:331–6.
5. Sinha V, Ramasamy R. Post-vasectomy pain syndrome: diagnosis, management and treatment options. Transl Androl Urol. 2017;6(Suppl 1):S44–7.
6. Maatman TJ, Aldrin L, Carothers GG. Patient noncompliance after vasectomy. Fertil Steril. 1997;68:552–5.
7. Murphy R, Perkins A, Marks MB, Burrows PJ, Marks SF. Post Vasectomy Reversal Semen Analysis Compliancy. Androl. 2012;33(Suppl2):42.

8. Teerawattananon C, Tantayakom P, Suwanawiboon B, Katchamart W. Risk of perioperative bleeding related to highly selective cyclooxygenase-2 inhibitors: A systematic review and meta-analysis. Semin Arthritis Rheum. 2017;46(4):520–8.
9. Drobnis EZ, Nangia AK. Male Reproductive Functions Disrupted by Pharmacological Agents. Adv Exp Med Biol. 2017;1034:13–24.
10. Rao M, Zhao XL, Yang J, Hu SF, Lei H, Xia W, Zhu CH. Effect of transient scrotal hyperthermia on sperm parameters, seminal plasma biochemical markers, and oxidative stress in men. Asian J Androl. 2015;17(4):668–75.
11. Alom M, Ziegelmann M, Savage J, Miest T, Köhler TS, Trost L. Office-based andrology and male infertility procedures-a cost-effective alternative. Transl Androl Urol. 2017;6(4):761–72.

Chapter 5
Vasectomy Reversal: The First Steps

Performing a correctly performed microsurgical vasectomy reversal is so much more than throwing a few microsutures. There are a number of preparations the surgeon should take as well as key concepts before and during the reversal to ensure that the patient receives the very best care and surgical outcomes. This chapter highlights some of the critical steps and how we work through challenges in our program before and during the pre-anastomosis portion of a vasovasostomy or vasoepididymostomy. Confirming that the OR has all that you will need before you start the reversal ensures that there will be no surprises. It is important to understand crucial principals about preserving the tissues, locating the vasal defect, confirming abdominal patency, and transecting the vas. Analysis of the vasal fluid, both gross and microscopic, guides the intraoperative decision-making as to whether to perform a vasovasostomy or vasoepididymostomy. Challenges often occur with indeterminate vasal fluid with concerns about cross contamination. Sperm banking during the reversal is an option to be discussed preoperatively with the patient.

Confirm Before You Start

Before each and every case, especially at surgery centers and hospitals, it is important to confirm with your OR circulator that they have available and ready all of the critical microinstruments, enough specific microsutures and whatever else may be necessary for you to perform the reversal that day. It is smart before you start to also confirm backup light bulbs are available for the surgical microscope and lab scope. If you have performed reversals long enough at a variety of centers, you will most likely have been halfway through a reversal when the circulating nurse announces that they have run out of the specific microsuture that you just asked for and that you routinely use, offering you instead something similar that they think should be fine (and rarely is). If intraoperative sperm banking is an option, you should have the special prep ready, such as a vial of HTF (human tubule fluid/sperm

© Springer Nature Switzerland AG 2019
S. H. F. Marks, *Vasectomy Reversal*,
https://doi.org/10.1007/978-3-030-00455-2_5

washing medium, Irvine Scientific, Catalog ID 9983), and confirm that the andrologist is there on-site and ready to accept the specimens. Finally, verify that the OR has your vasoepididymostomy microinstrument tray and microsutures ready, if needed, even if the patient has a short obstructive interval from vasectomy and you anticipate a VV.

Prophylactic Antibiotics

We routinely give all patients perioperative prophylactic broad-spectrum antibiotics – cephalexin (Kefzol) 1 gram IV – to prevent infection. Though the risks for infection are rare in a "clean-contaminated" wound and many experts do not use prophylactic antibiotics unless the patients are considered high risk [1–3], any intra-scrotal infection can be devastating to the patient, disastrous for the success of the reversal, and make any future surgery or a redo reversal attempt especially difficult.

Vasovasostomy: Pre-anastomosis

As you begin the reversal, there are a number of key steps before the surgery begins and then to retrieve and prepare the vas before the anastomosis. Taking the time to address these points will allow for easier surgery with fewer problems and better results.

Pre-reversal Exam

Once the patient is adequately sedated or asleep under general anesthesia, it is smart to perform a scrotal exam, before or after the prep and drape, to better assess the patient's specific anatomy and any post-vasectomy findings. You will get much more information with a better exam when the patient is sedated or asleep than you can preoperatively. This allows you to evaluate the vasal gaps for their location in the spermatic cord, the length of the gaps, possible clips or ties, the presence of a sperm granuloma, and, if present, the size, as well as other pathology. This can include thickening of the cord with induration from a prior bleed, infection, or failed prior reversal attempt, epididymal cysts, and the presence of a hydrocele or a tes-ticular or spermatic cord mass. This is when you will get the most information from an examination of the testicle for any pathology, peri-testicular scarring from prior surgery, any atrophic changes, masses, or evidence of prior trauma. This added information will allow you to more precisely plan the surgical approach and the incisions and anticipate and address any anatomic or surgical issues or concerns that may impact on the reversal.

Local Anesthesia

We infiltrate about 10 cc of local anesthetic solution into the scrotal skin along the planned incision site and underlying subcutaneous tissues before we start, even if the patient is under general anesthesia. We have found we achieve the best results with a 1:1 solution of 2% plain lidocaine and 0.5% plain bupivacaine. Once we have made the incision, we instill more local anesthetic high in the proximal spermatic cord and peri-vasal tissues. It is important to take care not to inject the local into the vas itself. If the incision must be extended, then infiltrate additional local along the anticipated incision path. Providing a cord block before addressing the vas and performing the reversal ensures that patient remains comfortable and pain-free during and after the procedure.

Incision Options

Most reversals are performed using a single midline vertical scrotal incision or two lateral vertical scrotal incisions (Fig. 5.1). Though there are advantages to both, we have found that most often the technique preferred by each surgeon is the approach learned in their residency or fellowship training.

When considering the length of the incision, in general it is best to use the smallest incision or incisions possible that will allow for adequate access and visualization of the damaged vas. Most often a 3–4 cm incision is fine. Wherever the incision(s), you should allow for possible extension as warranted by the intra-op findings and possible need for delivery of the testicle for a vasoepididymostomy or extended abdominal peri-vasal dissection. In my practice, I have found that a single midline incision provides plenty of access almost all the time whether for a VE or for more proximal exploration. If, at the time of the pre-reversal exam, I have concerns about a high abdominal vas or lengthy gaps, then I will use lateral vertical scrotal incisions. Dr. Peter Burrows here at our center prefers the two lateral vertical incisions.

Some experts prefer to use the mini-incision technique as proposed by Dr. Keith Jarvi, which for selected cases may be a viable option [4–6]. Each side must be assessed for anatomy and post-vasectomy changes to determine the size and location of incision(s) and if a mini-incision is appropriate. If the mini-incision approach is found to be inadequate, then the incision can be extended as needed. The concern with the mini-incision approach is that it is important to be careful not to make incision too small, which could limit direct visualization of the vas and peri-vasal

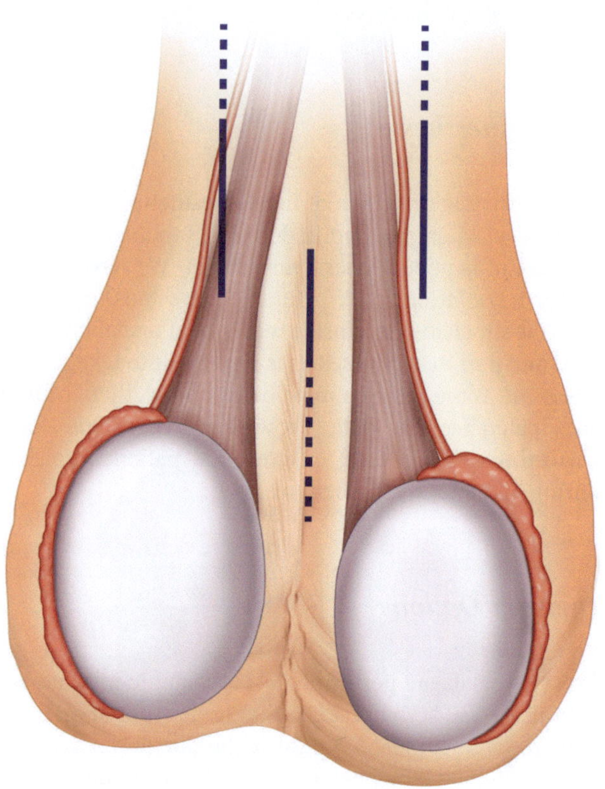

Fig. 5.1 Most experts use either a single vertical midline scrotal incision or two lateral vertical scrotal incisions

tissues, and so theoretically increase the risk for missing a bleeding vessel. Though a small incision is very appealing to patients, I have only had one patient in more than 3 decades, and many thousands of reversals complain that the 3 cm scrotal incision that we used was too long.

Finding the Vasectomy Site

Palpate the entire length of the vas superiorly to inferiorly, between the thumb and forefinger, gently feeling for a gap, metal clips, ties, or subtle thinning or thickening to identify and localize the damaged portion of the vasectomy site or adherent scar or fat. Usually this is easy to find. Often the only sign is dense or vascular changes in the peri-vasal tissues overlying the vasectomy location.

If You Are Unable to Identify the Vasectomy Site

On rare occasions the vasal defect or scar from the vasectomy might not be identified. If no palpable irregularity or deformity is easily identified, then visually look at the length of the vas through the surgical microscope for any remnants of any vasectomy sutures that may be present. Sometimes pinpoint black or blue dots are a clue that may represent residual sutures. Other times you can see an amber dot or nodule of an absorbable suture. Another trick is to look for the localization of any fat or adventitia that may be adherent to the vas. If this fat is gently teased off the vas, often you can see remnants of ties or of the damaged vas that was otherwise felt to be intact. Sometimes we have been surprised to find the vasectomy site much further down in the very deep convoluted vas or even a small wedge of the tail of the epididymis excised. What makes this even more challenging is that the vasectomy on the contralateral side may have been performed where most vasectomies are usually located up in the mid straight vas.

If the vasectomy site is still not localized, we have found that if you deliver the testicle, if not already done, this may allow you to find the vasectomy site if very low deep in the convoluted vas or distal epididymis. You may need to open the tunica vaginalis for examination of the distal epididymis. Other times, we have found the vasectomy site very high up in the scrotum, just below the inguinal canal (Fig. 5.2). It may a good idea at this point to move over to the contralateral side and see if the vasectomy site can be identified there. If so, then repair that side and return to the initial side, knowing what to look for.

If you are still unable to localize the vasectomy site, and the patient has a known history of hernia repair, orchiopexy, torsion, or any inguinal or pelvic surgery, then we presume that the vasectomy was performed in the groin or pelvis concomitantly with the other inguinal or pelvic/abdominal surgery [7–10]. It is important to realize this concern is not just with pelvic surgeries, as we have had a patient that had an intra-abdominal laparoscopic vasectomy at the time of elective cholecystectomy. Another patient had a laparoscopic vasectomy on one side when his hernia was repaired and a transscrotal vasectomy through a midline incision on the other, so the patient, not understanding, thought the vasectomy was performed transscrotally on both sides. At this point we rereview the medical records and also closely reexamine the patient for an inguinal incision to see if the vasectomy may have been performed inguinally. With so many inguinal hernias repaired laparoscopically, alone or concomitantly with other pelvic or abdominal surgery, there are instances when there is no identifiable vasectomy site, no inguinal scar and no history of hernia repair. This is when we or the nurse would talk to the partner, if available, to see if she might be aware of any abdominal or inguinal surgery that they forgot to mention.

Very rarely, you may not be able to find the vasectomy site. If you are unable to identify the vasectomy site on one or both sides, then you have several options. You may perform the reversal only on the contralateral side where you are able to

Fig. 5.2 The transscrotal vasectomy site can be very low, deep in the convoluted vas or even within the distal epididymis or very high in the scrotum, almost subinguinal

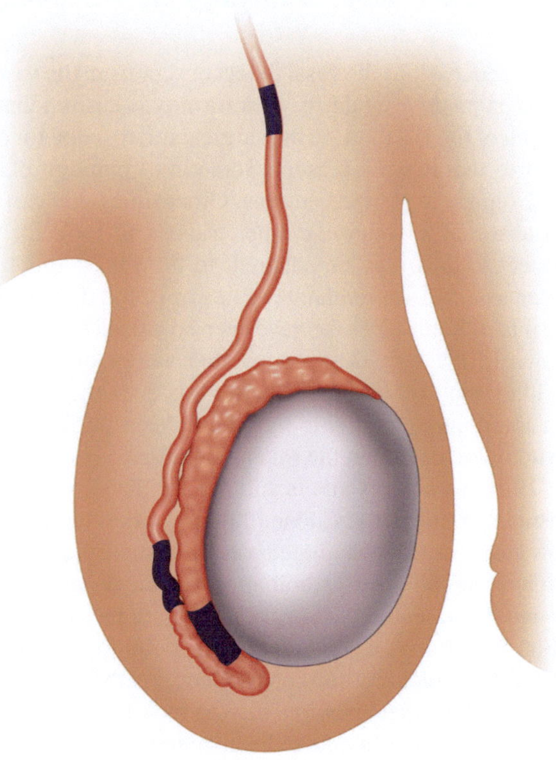

localize the vasectomy site and then in the future discuss options if the post-unilateral reversal results are not adequate. Another is to not proceed with the reversal at that time and instead advise the patient that a laparoscopic evaluation is indicated and either reschedule or refer to an expert experienced in robotic laparoscopic vasovasostomies. Another is to make an "educated guess" based on your experience where you think the vasectomy was performed and assess the patency of the abdominal and testicular vas to see if there is any proximal or distal obstruction that might localize the vasectomy site. If the abdominal vas on the contralateral side is open and healthy but there is epididymal obstruction, with known or presumed inguinal obstruction and no epididymal blockage on the ipsilateral side, it may be reasonable to perform a transseptal crossover where the long abdominal segment of the contralateral vas is brought over through the septum and anastomosed to the testicular vas above the healthy testicle and open epididymis [11, 12] (Fig. 5.3).

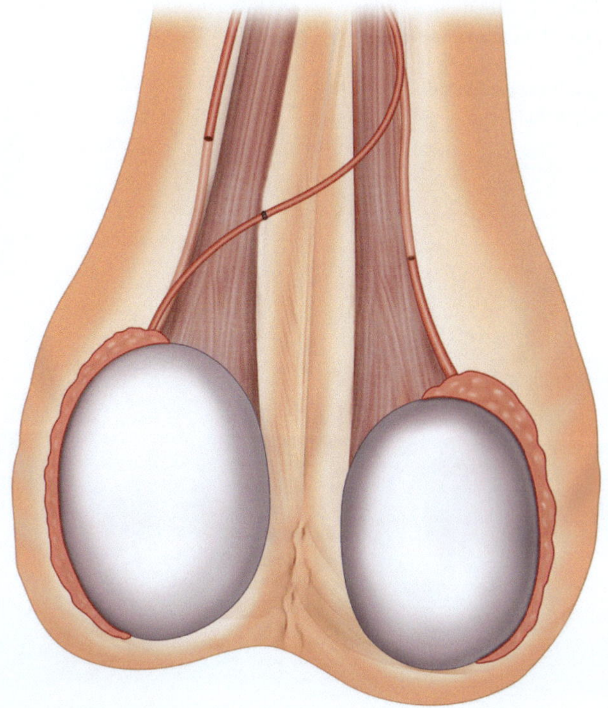

Fig. 5.3 A transseptal vasovasostomy with the long abdominal vas brought through the septum to be anastomosed to the contralateral testicular vas

Once the Vasectomy Site Is Localized

Evaluate the vas and defect for important information, to include the length of the vasal gap, extent of vasal damage and scar, presence and location of metal clips or ties, as well as possible calcifications in the vas. Though most often the vasal gap is one or two cm in length, there are occasions you may encounter a 5–7 cm gap between the abdominal and testicular vas. Many times, we have found that the actual extent of vasal damage from the vasectomy was much more than what would have been predicted by the pre-op palpation of the vasal gap. This can be from vasal damage from placement of metal clips across the vas many centimeters above and below the excised segment (Fig. 5.4) or from excessive intravasal or peri-vasal cautery at the time of the vasectomy (Fig. 5.5) or scarring from other intrascrotal surgery or trauma, post-reversal peri-vasal bleeding, hematoma, or infection.

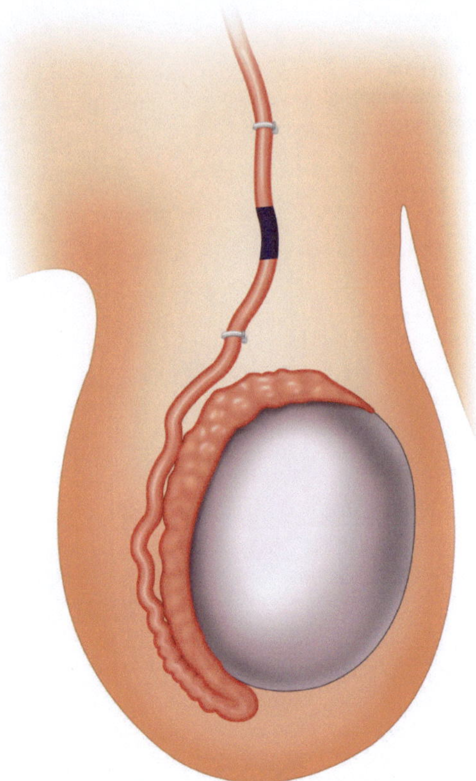

Fig. 5.4 Metal clips placed on the vas several cm above and below the small excised vasal segment

Delivery of the Vasectomy Site

There are two schools of thought when it comes to delivery of the vasectomy site through the incision. The first approach and the one that I use is to simply deliver just the portion of the vas that contains the vasectomy site so that it looks like strand of spaghetti looping out of a button hole. The other technique is to deliver the entire hemiscrotal contents (cord and testicle) on that side. Of course, it's about what works best for you and your patient.

Delivery of Just the Vas

Once you have identified the vasectomy site, then it is usually very simple to deliver and excise the portion of the vas that contains the vasectomy scar with enough vas to be able to easily perform the repair (Fig. 5.6). Then, if you need to proceed with a vasoepididymostomy, it is easy to extend the incision inferiorly as much as needed so that you can deliver the testicle. Most often the small incision is enough to bring out the testicle for the VE.

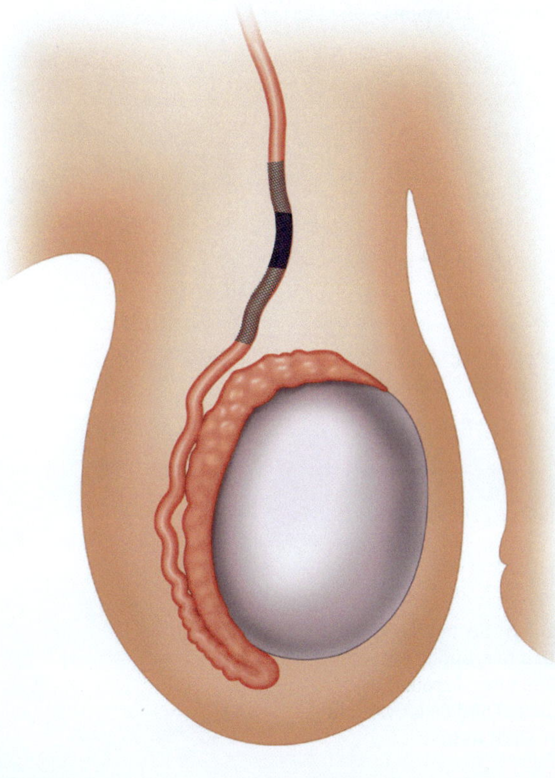

Fig. 5.5 Excessive vasal scarring proximal and distal to the vasectomy gap presumed from excessive intravasal or peri-vasal cautery

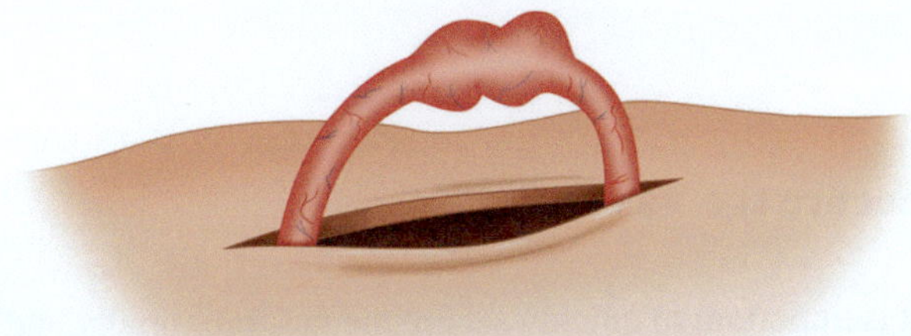

Fig. 5.6 Delivery of just the vasectomy site and adjacent healthy vas out of the incision

Delivery of the Hemiscrotal Contents

There are other reversal experts that prefer to deliver the hemiscrotal contents on each side, leaving the tunica vaginalis intact unless access to the epididymis is needed (Fig. 5.7). They feel that this approach provides for better visualization of the vas and testicle and allows for easier access to the epididymis for evaluation and/ or vasoepididymostomy.

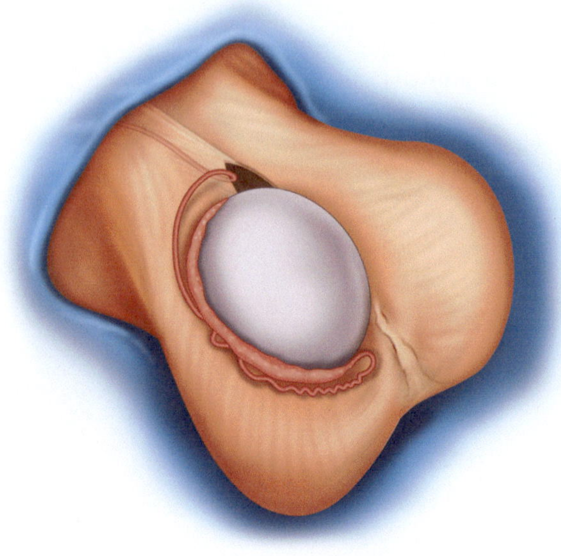

Fig. 5.7 Delivery of entire hemiscrotal contents

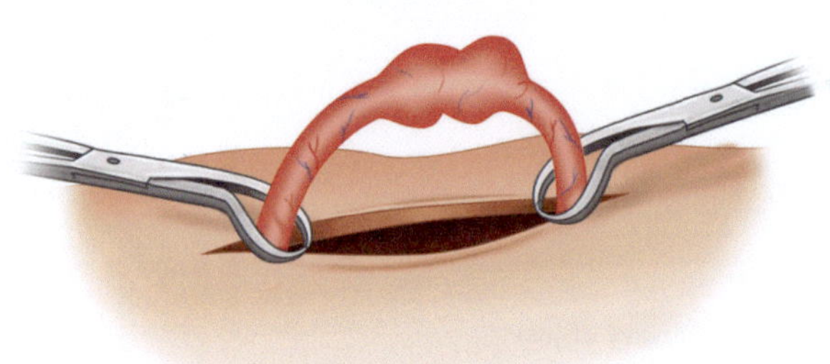

Fig. 5.8 Secure the vas with a fine-tipped towel clamp placed around the proximal and distal vas and peri-vasal tissues

Secure the Vas

It is important to quickly secure the vas, proximally and distally, prior to transection of the vas. I have found that fine-tipped sharp towel clamps work well in my practice to secure the vas, placed around the vas and peri-vasal tissues as far up and down the spermatic cord as you can (Fig. 5.8). Be careful to place the points of towel clamps behind the vas under direct vision to avoid inadvertently damaging any underlying peri-vasal vessels. Then, when the secured vas is transected, the cut ends of the vas won't retract and pull back deep inguinally or down to the testicle. If the vas is not properly secured and does pull away and retracts deeply, this can force you to go "hunting" for the transected end. This can be especially challenging if a small vessel is actively bleeding and distorting the normal anatomy, making localization and retrieval of the retracted vas more difficult. We then leave these securing towel clamps in place throughout the reversal and remove them only after the anastomosis is complete, and we have verified there is no bleeding.

Preserve and Protect the Peri-vasal Blood Supply

Absolutely no cautery should be used directly on or near the vas. Only use bipolar to control vasal bleeding and never on the transected face of the vas or at the lumen. Small peri-vasal vessels can be tied with nonabsorbable suture such as 5–0 to 7–0 nylon. It is best to avoid using absorbable sutures on or adjacent to the vas as the tissue reaction and inflammatory reabsorption process of the suture material may generalize into adjacent tissues and the vas and so theoretically might increase the risks for intravasal inflammation and scarring.

Do Not Skeletonize the Vas

Do not skeletonize the vas by peeling back or removing the adventitia to expose a "cleaner," more pristine vas in preparation for transection. To maintain the critical vasal blood supply, it is critical to allow the adventitial tissues to remain intact and adherent to the vas right up to the transected face throughout the reversal. Quite often when we perform a redo reversal, we encounter a nonviable, atretic segment of vas above and/or below the anastomosis site, which is consistent with a compromised blood supply to the ends of the vas at the time of the failed first repair. This will make an easier and more aesthetically pleasing repair but actually increases risks for ischemic scarring from devascularization.

The Microblade

Microblades used to transect the vas are extremely sharp and delicate, so they often become dull after just two or three passes through the vas. To ensure a smooth transection of the vas with minimal trauma, replace the blades frequently, especially if you inadvertently drag the blade across a metal clip. A dull blade causes more trauma as it tears and shears rather than slices cleanly through the vas. Be careful as some of the stainless steel microblades can be very brittle and easily break into multiple small pieces, which are difficult to find in the open wound. Do not try to force a blade that is too thick through the guide slot. Before you insert a microblade into the guide slot of the vas cutting forceps, inspect the blade under the surgical microscope to confirm that the blade is clean without any adherent debris, dried blood clots, or irregularities along the cutting edge. These can cause snagging or dragging of the blade as it is drawn though the vas, which can lead to an irregular, ragged transection of the vas.

There are a few tricks that can reduce costs and ensure that you have the sharpest blades. One is to cut the long 35 mm straight microblade (ASSI.CBS35) in half with standard heavy bandage scissors (Fig. 5.9). Instead of having one long blade,

Fig. 5.9 Cut the microblade in half with heavy scissors to provide two blades, each with a fresh cutting surfaces on either end. (Photo Credit: Sheldon Marks)

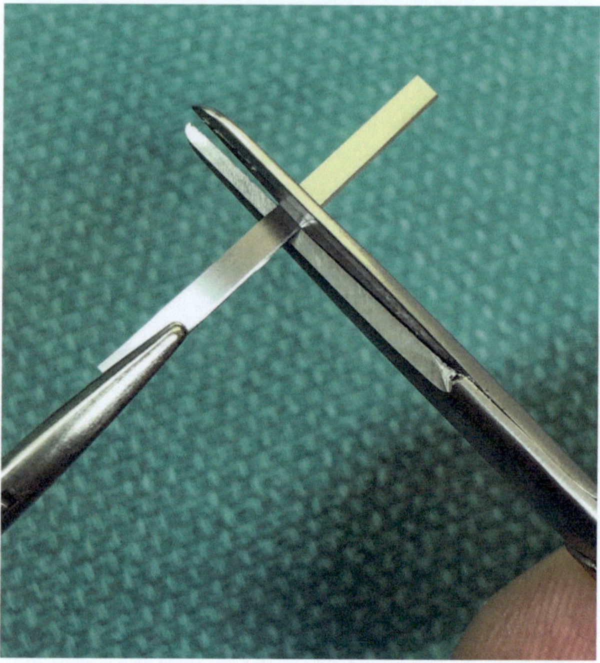

now you have two halves, and each half can be used twice on each side for a total of four to six passes per half. After two passes on the first side, simply flip and secure the half blade in the blade holder (ASSI.BHS12), and you can usually use the unused half for the second side. This allows you to cut your costs so that in most instances you can use only ½ of a microblade for the entire reversal. If you find that you do need another blade, then the other half will already be sterilized and available. A second trick to have incredibly sharp blades and save even more money is to use a standard "old-fashioned" safety razor blade and simply cut off the long, thin connecting segments with heavy bandage scissors (Fig. 5.10). We have had very good results with this technique at a fraction of the cost of the standard surgical microblades.

Transection of the Vas

Transecting the vas above and below the vasectomy scar is not just cutting out the damaged vas and scar. It is critical to use the right tools with the best techniques to minimize trauma and ensure the ideal anatomy to make the technical anastomosis easier and minimize complications. These are the techniques, tips, and tricks we use when preparing the vas for the repair.

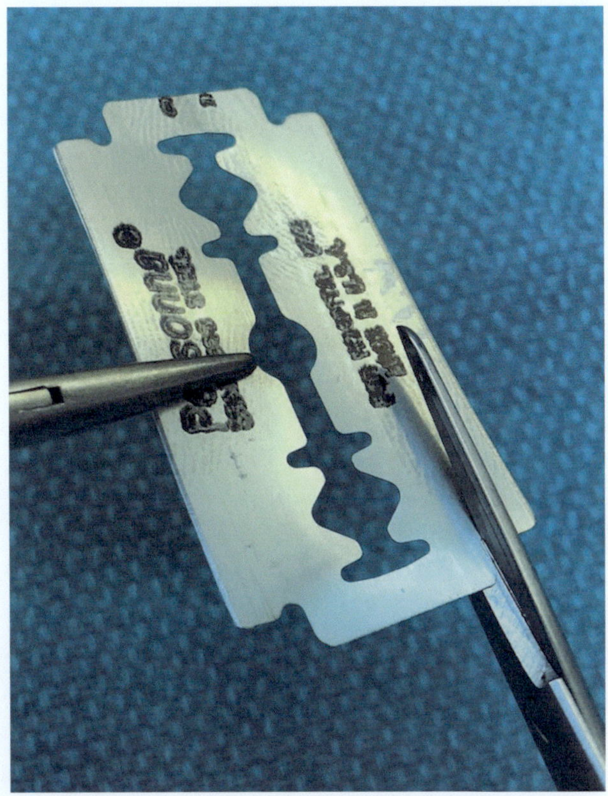

Fig. 5.10 Use heavy scissors to cut out the central arms of a safety razor blade, providing two long blades. (Photo Credit: Sheldon Marks)

Vas Cutting Forceps: Angled, Straight, or 11 Blade

The goal is to achieve a smooth, cleanly cut face of the vas to allow for a more precise coaptation of the abdominal and testicular vas. There are the options most top reversal experts use to hold and transect the vas. The most common three are:

1. Angled Marks Vas Cutting Forceps (ASSI.NHF-2.15, 2.5.15 or 3.15)
2. 90° blade slot vas/nerve holding forceps (ASSI.NHF-2, 2.5, or 3)
3. #11 scalpel blade over 6-inch sterile wood tongue depressor

Most experts prefer the use of a vas cutting forceps (also called a nerve holding clamp) (Fig. 5.11) with a fresh Dennis, Beaver, or similar microblade through the eccentrically located blade slot. This technique offers a more precise transection of the vas, which is held securely in place so there is less shearing and crushing trauma to the vas than with the use of a thicker 11 blade, where the vas is compressed down as it is cut over a sterile wood tongue depressor.

The angled Marks Vas Cutting Forceps with a 15° blade guide slot (Fig. 5.12) was developed with a leading expert in wound healing to create a slightly larger

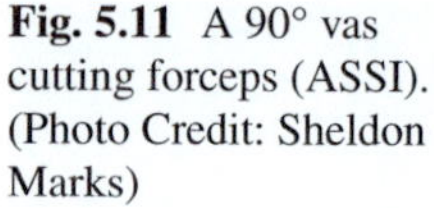

Fig. 5.11 A 90° vas cutting forceps (ASSI). (Photo Credit: Sheldon Marks)

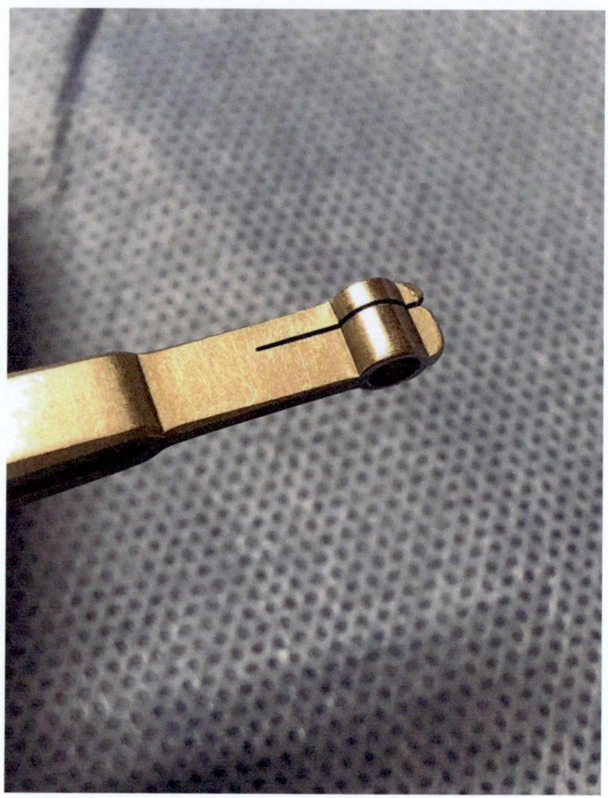

elliptical lumen of the vas and so increase the surface area rather than round lumen obtained with a standard right-angle transection [13]. A recent review demonstrated that the angled vas cutting forceps provides a higher success with reduced anastomotic stricturing and obstruction, presumed to be from larger elliptical lumen. When you use the angled vas cutting forceps, note the instrument labeling on the side of the forceps facing the surgeon to be replicated on the second vasal transection. This then ensures that the angled cut faces of the vas are aligned to maximize the approximation of the lumens (Figs. 5.13 and 5.14).

Positioning of the Vas Cutting Forceps

Place the vas cutting forceps over the entire vas, including the peri-vasal adventitia. This should be positioned in its natural orientation and on no traction within several mm just above or below the vasectomy site and any metal clips, in what feels and appears to be normal smooth vas, free of scarring and induration (Fig. 5.15). Confirm that the vas is mobilized enough so that when secured, the vas can be easily rotated at least 90° each way. When you transect the abdominal vas above the vasectomy

Fig. 5.12 The Marks angled vas cutting forceps by ASSI with a 15° blade slot to increase the elliptical surface area of the lumen. (Photo Credit: Sheldon Marks)

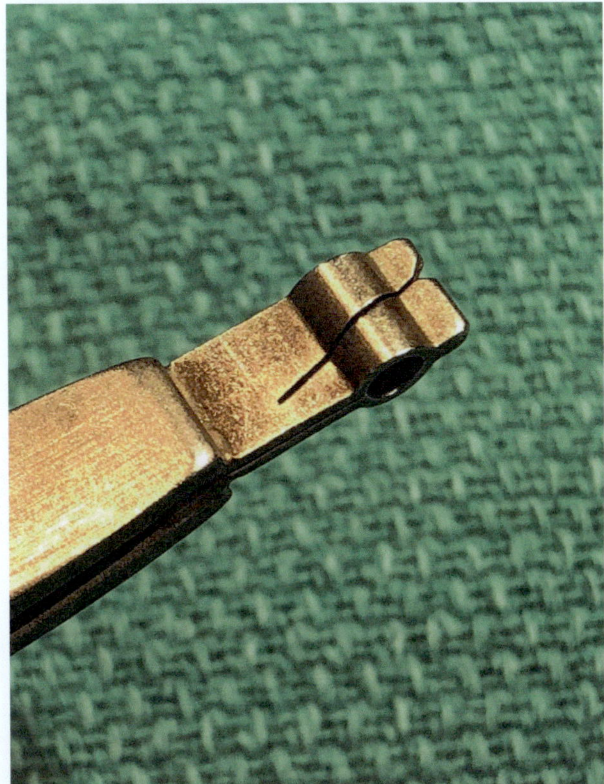

Fig. 5.13 Confirm that the same instrument labeling is always facing the surgeon when transecting both the abdominal and testicular vas so the angled of the face of the vas is consistent on both sides. (Photo Credit: Sheldon Marks)

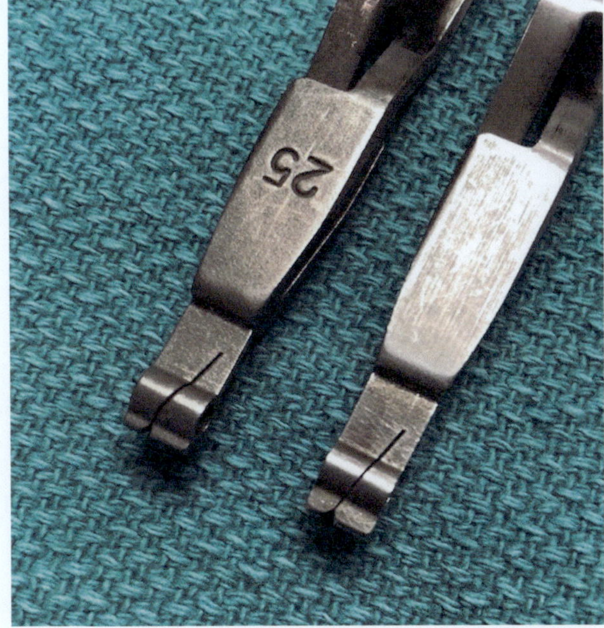

Fig. 5.14 Alignment of both the abdominal and testicular transected vas to maximize the increase elliptical lumen size

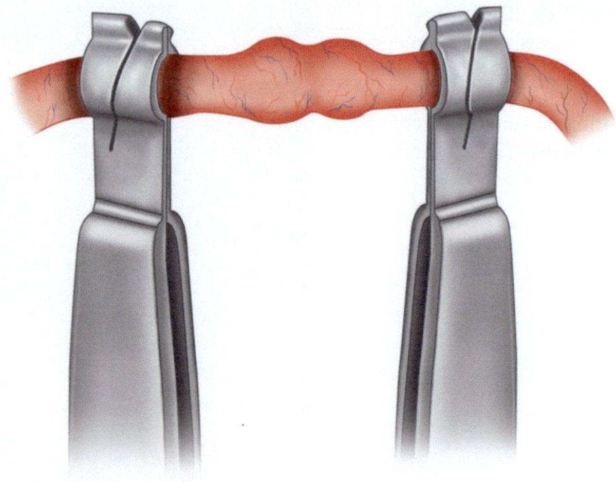

Fig. 5.15 Place the vas cutting forceps onto the vas several mm from the damaged vas, on no traction

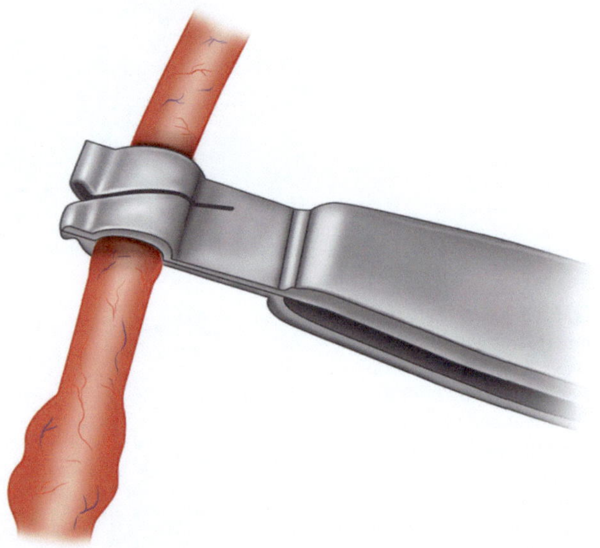

scar, preserve as much vasal length as possible. The challenge is to be as close to the vasal defect as you can to ensure the transection is in healthy vas without any vasal damage or scarring from the vasectomy. Be sure the vas cutting forceps are holding the vas at a 90° angle to the line of the vas when you pass the blade (Fig. 5.16). Identify and do not include any large peri-vasal blood vessels in the vas cutting forceps.

Transecting the Vas

Under direct vision through the surgical microscope, insert the clean blade all the way through the top of the guide slot in the vas cutting forceps, above the vas, to the hilt of the blade holder (Fig. 5.17). If there is dense or especially thick peri-vasal adventitia, then you can also pass the blade up into the forceps guide slot from the open side. Having all three sizes of the slotted vas cutting forceps, 2.0, 2.5, and 3.0 will allow you to use the most appropriate vas cutting forceps that best fits the diameter of the vas (Fig. 5.18). Pull the blade with a gentle but firm downward minimal

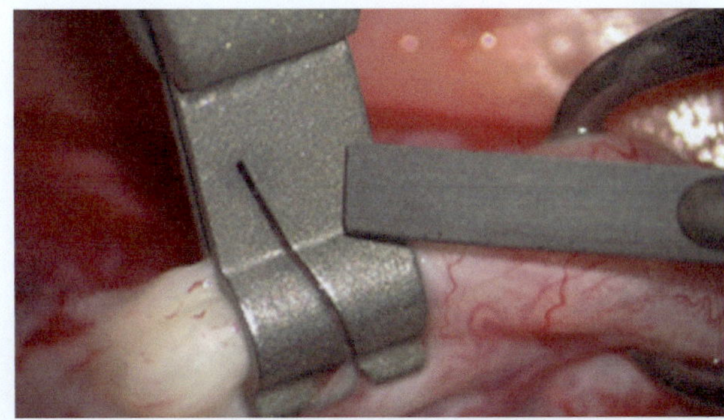

Fig. 5.16 Hold the vas cutting forceps at a right angle to the vas, avoiding any large peri-vasal blood vessels. (Photo Credit: Sheldon Marks)

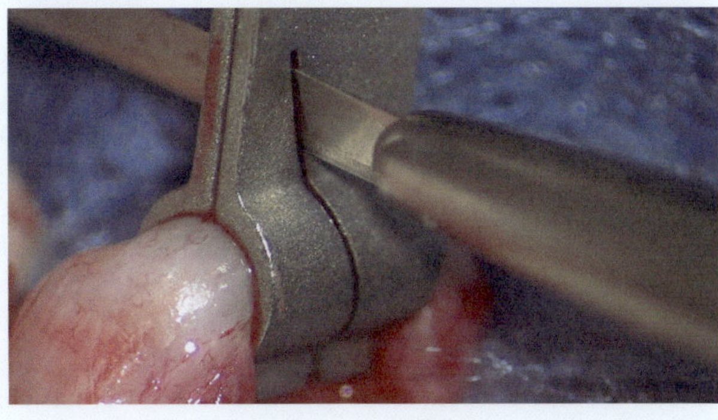

Fig. 5.17 Microblade is inserted completely into the top of the blade slot. (Photo Credit: Sheldon Marks)

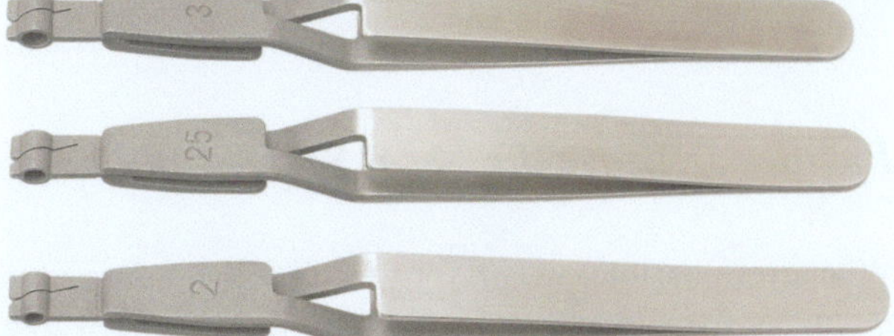

Fig. 5.18 Use the most appropriate of the three sizes of the Marks angled vas cutting forceps, 2.0, 2.5, and 3.0. (Photo Credit: Accurate Surgical and Scientific Instruments, Corp. [ASSI])

Fig. 5.19 With a single pass, draw the microblade toward the surgeon with gentle downward pressure. (Photo Credit: Sheldon Marks)

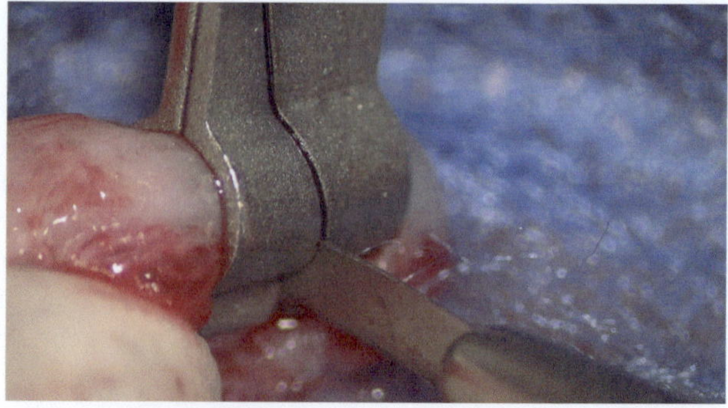

Fig. 5.20 Grasp the transected edge of the peri-vasal adventitia with microhemostat. (Photo Credit: Sheldon Marks)

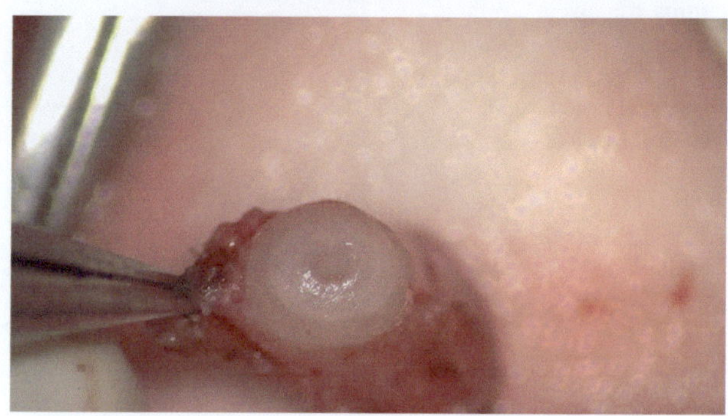

pressure as you draw the blade toward yourself. Avoid a sawing, back-and-forth rocking motion (Fig. 5.19). This should be easy to do with a single pass when using a fresh, clean blade. If the blade only partially transects the vas or you feel a scraping, dragging sensation, then this tells you that the blade is dull or that you are cutting through scar or up against a metal clip. Replace with a new blade and recut the vas 1 or 2 mm over after you clean the blade guide slot to wash away any debris or clots.

After you have passed the blade, immediately grasp and secure the edge of the cut adventitia with the tip of a microhemostat (Fig. 5.20). Then take a moment to look through the surgical microscope at the small peri-vasal and adventitial blood vessels around the transected the vas as these vessels can be inadvertently partially incised or totally cut when the blade is passed. If any vessels have been cut, then tie or use bipolar to control any bleeding.

Remove or Leave the Vasal Scar/Granuloma

Whenever possible, we prefer to excise the damaged vasectomy scar and adjacent remnants. We always excise a sperm granuloma with any scar rather than leaving this inflammatory mass in place, adjacent to the new repair. Care must be taken removing a granuloma as often there may be significantly increased vascularity in the peri-granuloma tissues. The only reason to bypass and leave the damaged vas in place is when there is multiple large blood vessels coursing through dense, peri-vasal scar or if there is a lengthy segment of very minimal scar in the gap between the ends of the vas (Fig. 5.21).

Examine the Transected Face and Vasal Lumen

Knowing what to look for after transecting the vas will significantly improve the ease and success of the anastomosis. Taking the time to be sure that transected vas is not still in scar or that the lumen is not ideal will make passing of the microsutures easier with fewer problems.

What's the Goal?

After the vas is transected, it is important to closely examine the face of the abdominal and testicular vas through the surgical microscope to be sure that you have a clean, healthy vasal face with no scarring or irregularities. The goal is a centrally located lumen with round, symmetric "bulls-eye" muscularis layers with a clean mucosal edge clearly defined (Fig. 5.22). Then examine the vasal lumen to be sure that the mucosal edge is visible, clean, and healthy appearing. If needed, you should be able to easily place the tip of microforceps just inside the lumen and gently open to better visualize a mm or 2 up inside the lumen (Fig. 5.23). You can use this

Fig. 5.21 Vasal remnant with minimal scar can be bypassed

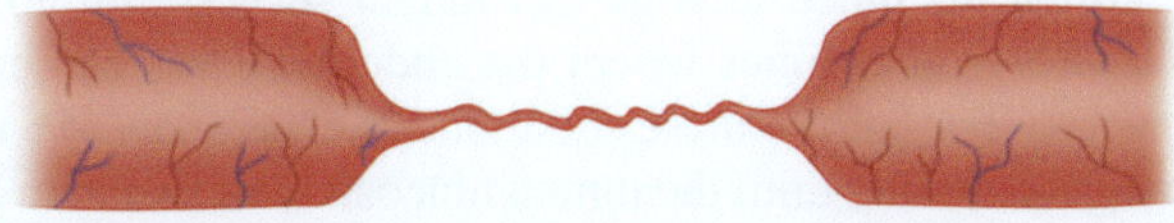

Fig. 5.22 The goal is a centrally located lumen with round, symmetric "bulls-eye" muscularis layers with a clean mucosal edge clearly defined. (Photo Credit: Sheldon Marks)

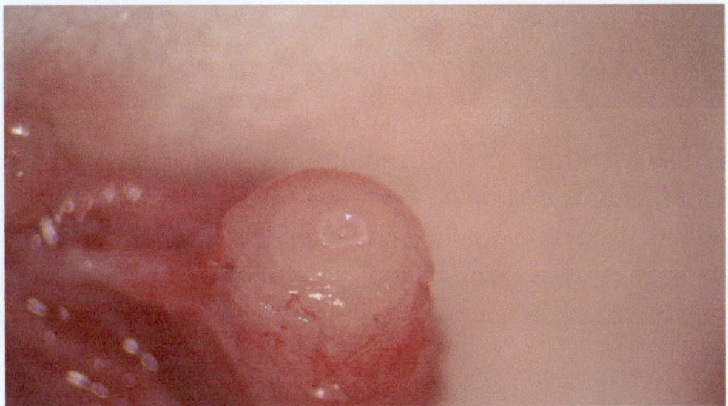

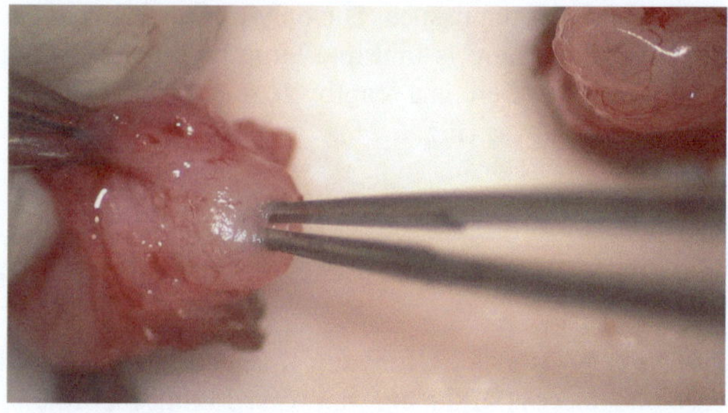

Fig. 5.23 Insert the tip of the microforceps just inside the lumen and gently open to better visualize a mm or 2 up inside the lumen. (Photo Credit: Sheldon Marks)

technique to better visualize the lumen and mucosal edge and provide countertraction when passing the luminal 70 or 100 micron needle.

Do Not Dilate the Lumen

It is not wise to forcibly dilate the lumen with lacrimal dilators or forceps. In fact, there is really no reason to use lacrimal dilators. This old technique is unnecessary and should be abandoned as it causes stretching, tearing, and microtrauma to the delicate luminal mucosa and so potentially increased risks for subsequent scarring. If the lumen is felt to be too tight from scar or because the transection is too close to the damaged portion of the vas, then the solution is to re-resect the vas a few mm more proximally or distally. It is acceptable to use the tips of the microforceps barely inserted into the lumen to gently separate the edges and allow for better visualization of the luminal edge when passing the needles. Sometimes you will find that the mucosal edge can retract several mm up into the abdominal lumen. There are other times where the abdominal vas can have a protruding, "pouchy" mucosa. For both of these situations, the vas should be recut a few mm more proximally or distally until the lumen mucosa is clean and in line with the transected face of the vas.

If the Vas Is Scarred or Irregular

If there is scarring or irregularity of the muscularis or if the transected vas is not ideal, then it is wise to recut the vas superiorly or inferiorly an additional 1–2 mm, again based on palpable and visual findings (Fig. 5.24). Continue to transect the vas, and reexamine through the microscope until a clean, smooth vas with a healthy bulls-eye appearance with central lumen and clean mucosal edge is visible.

Fig. 5.24 Irregular or scarred transected face of the vas

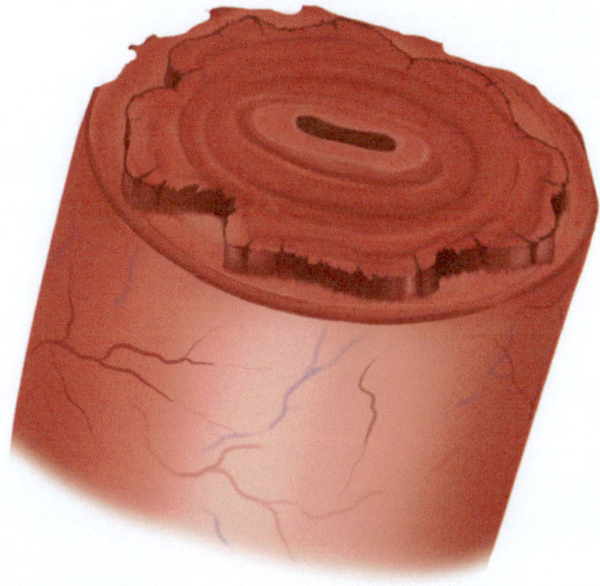

Fig. 5.25 Eccentric vasal lumen

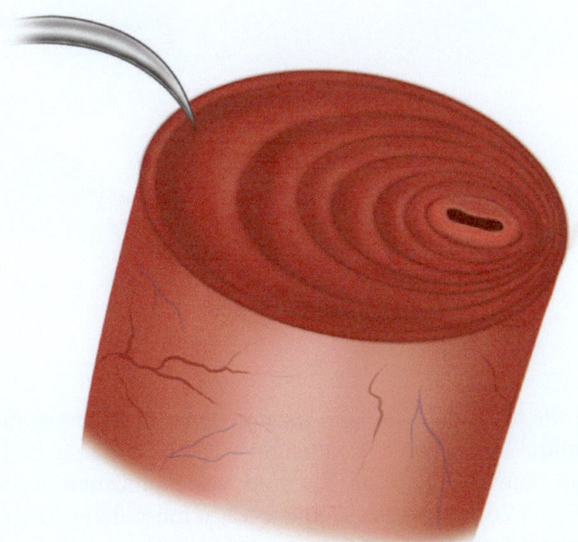

Eccentric Lumen/Convoluted Vas

If an eccentric, angled lumen is seen, the vas should be retransected as this often has a thin overlying portion of the muscularis (Fig. 5.25). It may take several transections of the vas to find a more centrally located lumen. If the vas is convoluted and has a very thin wall on one side, then recut until you have a more central lumen.

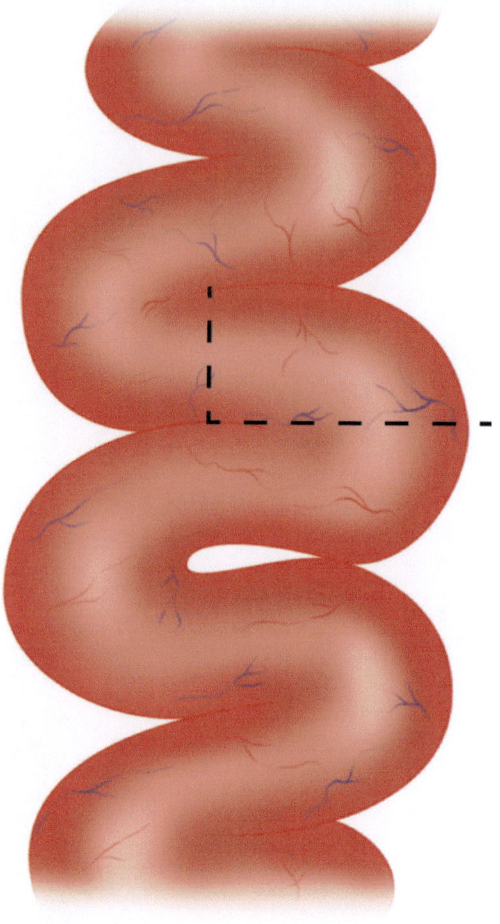

Fig. 5.26 Transect at the apex of the arch in the convoluted vas or along the straight portion in between the arches in convoluted vas to find a more centrally located lumen

If the testicular side is in located down in the convoluted vas, then finding a good central lumen can be challenging. It is best to transect the vas at the apex of arch of the convolution or in the mid vas equidistant from the two arching portions (Fig. 5.26). If there is adequate vasal muscularis around the lumen, then a less than central lumen may be acceptable [14, 15].

Confirm Abdominal Patency

The most common technique to confirm abdominal vasal patency is with a saline vasogram. To do this, cannulate the lumen of the abdominal vas through the surgical microscope with just the tip of a 24-gauge Angiocath on a 3 cc syringe. Gently instill 1–3 cc of heparinized saline or lactated Ringer's solution up into the lumen of

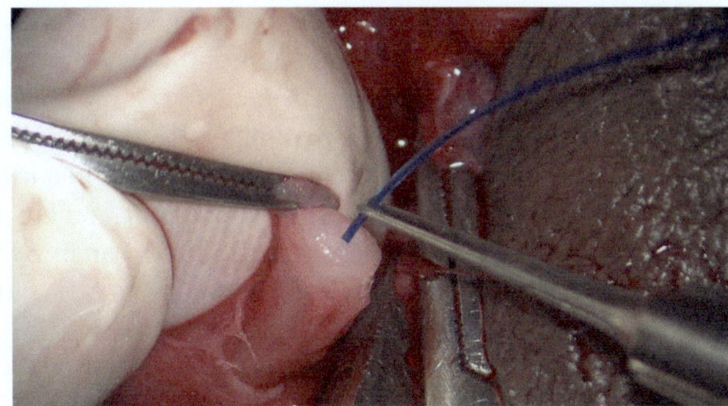

Fig. 5.27 Passing of the 0 polypropylene into the abdominal vas to identify the location of obstruction. (Photo Credit: Sheldon Marks)

the abdominal vas. If the fluid flows easily when instilled into the lumen, then this is presumptive evidence that the abdominal vas is open and not obstructed. Most often the fluid will flow easily. Do not forcibly push the fluid. There are times when the fluid will still flow, but more slowly.

If the fluid does not instill easily into the abdominal vas and instead sprays back when you try to introduce fluid into the lumen, this suggests a more proximal blockage such as in the groin or pelvis. We then gently pass the blunt end of a 0 polypropylene (Prolene®) up the lumen into the abdominal vas. Be careful to inspect the end of the polypropylene suture under the surgical microscope before you use it to be sure that it is not sharp or angled which might scrape and injure the delicate mucosa as it is passed up. If it is sharp, recut and smooth out the end of the polypropylene before it is inserted into the vas. If you encounter any obstruction when passing the suture so that the suture can't be passed any further, then we clamp a hemostat on the polypropylene where it enters the abdominal vas, withdraw the polypropylene, and measure the length of the suture from the hemostat to the end of the suture. We then place the length of polypropylene overlying the path of the vas up to localize the level of obstruction. Most often, in my experience, the blockage is usually in the inguinal region (Fig. 5.27).

There are other experts that prefer to perform a dye vasogram. They instill 2–3 ml of diluted indigo carmine in a 1:10 dilution into the abdominal vas via a 24-gauge Angiocath. After the dye is instilled into the vas, the bladder is catheterized, to obtain urine. The presence of blue to green urine verifies vasal patency. Repeating this on the second side adds the challenge of already having dye in the bladder from the previous vasogram on the first side. A formal radiographic vasogram, which is primarily beneficial before a robotic-assisted pelvic vasovasostomy to confirm and localize any obstruction, can be performed with 2–3 ml of diluted water-soluble contrast medium.

Vasal Fluid Analysis

Analysis of the vasal fluid is the most critical step that is often overlooked by many doctors that perform vasectomy reversals. The only correct way to decide whether to perform a VV or VE is with information from both the gross *and* microscopic vasal fluid analysis. It is not in the patient's best interests nor does it meet the standard of care for the surgeon to not appropriately assess the vasal fluid. Some doctors instead make assumptions based exclusively on the obstructive interval and the gross fluid alone or use other parameters as the justification for the reversal technique used. There are others that will only perform a bilateral VV on every patient. It is generally agreed by leading experts that if you are going to offer your patients a reversal, then you have the responsibility to analyze the vasal fluid microscopically to dictate whether to perform either VV or VE so that they receive the correct technique with the best possible chances for success.

Gross Fluid Findings

Look at and document the color, consistency, and volume of the vasal fluid from the testicular vasal lumen. Though the fluid usually remains the same, you may note that the color, consistency, and/or volume can change during the repair. For example, there are times when the fluid may be a mild volume initially and then, with time, the vasal fluid volume can increase and become moderate or even copious.

The vasal fluid volume is described as none, minimal, mild, moderate, and copious. I record the best fluid volume seen. We rate the vasal fluid color as clear, murky, white, yellow, or brown. Consistency of the vasal fluid is rated as watery, creamy, thick or paste-like. There are times when the fluid is more gel-like or even like crankcase oil. Some prefer to describe the fluid consistency as water-soluble or water insoluble. I cannot emphasize enough that the gross vasal fluid findings alone are not appropriate to use as the sole determinant for whether to perform a VV or VE. On occasion, you might initially find creamy white fluid that you will think is most likely consistent with a deeper epididymal obstruction, only to find whole sperm in the fluid microscopically. In the case of indeterminate microscopic findings, it is then appropriate to include the gross fluid findings as suggestive to help in your decision-making.

Preparing the Glass Slide

After the vas is transected, most often fluid will efflux from the testicular lumen. Simply dab the end of a sterile glass onto the transected face of the testicular vas to obtain a small drop of vasal fluid from the lumen. Quickly pass the slide to the circulating nurse to immediately apply a cover slip so that the drop does not dry out, which would still allow for sperm to be visualized but would prevent seeing any motility. As noted, oftentimes the first drop out of the vas is not representative of fluid that follows in gross or even microscopic findings. Do not be in such a hurry to only look at one slide if it is not favorable for a VV, which will have a higher chance for success than a VE. There are occasions when you will only see sperm debris, which during the anastomosis can progress to fluid with sperm with partial tails or even whole, motile sperm. I usually check several slides as the fluid starts to efflux if the first slides do not show adequate sperm or parts. To stay organized or if we need to look back at the slides, we attach to each slide a label with patient information and write on the slide with a Sharpie "right" or "left" and the number of slide, such as L1 or R4.

If the vasal fluid volume is minimal, then quickly add a small drop of heparinized saline, HTF, or LR to the drop of vasal fluid to keep it from drying out before the cover slip can be placed and the slide reviewed. If the vasal fluid is too creamy or thick, then we can add a small drop of irrigant and stir to dilute the fluid on the slide so that it becomes less dense, which makes it much easier to visualize any sperm that might be overlooked in the thicker specimen, dense with all the cellular debris. Another tip if there is no visible fluid at the lumen is to put a tiny drop of heparinized saline, HTF, or LR on the slide, and then touch this drop to testicular the end of the vas, as this will often pick up microscopic sperm. This absence of any vasal fluid is more common after excision of a sperm granuloma.

Techniques to Identify Sperm when None Are Seen in the Initial Vasal Fluid

1. *Review several consecutive slides* as sometimes sperm will be seen on subsequent slides even if none were present on the initial slides.
2. *Gentle milking* of the vas or even gentle distal epididymal compression may encourage fluid to efflux from testicular vas. Be aware that if there is a sperm granuloma, many times there will be only very minimal vasal fluid.
3. *Allow for time* to allow fluid deeper down to efflux from the vas. This can happen right away or may only start as you are tying the final mucosal sutures. There are occasions when I expect to see better results and so will pause that side and move to do the reversal on the contralateral side to allow for time to see if better fluid with sperm will be appear in the fluid.
4. *Gentle barbotage* of irrigant into the lumen via a 24-gauge Angiocath and then analyze the effluxing vasal fluid for sperm can show the presence of sperm when none were seen in the initial fluid.
5. *Sometimes small pulses* of room temperature irrigant onto the vas and epididymis can stimulate peristalsis of the testicular vas with increased flow of the vasal fluid now with whole sperm or sperm with long partial tails.

It is important to take your time and not be rushed, as the goal is to find the very best sperm that you can to drive you to perform a VV and if no whole sperm or parts are seen, then move to perform a VE. The surgeon or assistant would then review the slide under the adjacent lab microscope in the OR to look for sperm or sperm parts. Some doctors prefer to look at the slide themselves, while others use an andrologist. Then the circulator would pass the slide to the andrologist to analyze under their lab microscope, looking for sperm or sperm parts. On occasion, when the surgeon is unable to find sperm and so is considering performing a VE, the andrologist, who has the time and expertise to do a more comprehensive slide review, is able to identify rare whole and sometimes motile sperm or sperm with partial tails which directs us to perform the more successful vasovasostomy.

OR and Lab Microscope

Unless you have your own andrology lab, it is essential for the surgeon or assistant to examine the vasal or epididymal fluid to look for sperm or sperm parts to decide whether a VV or VE is indicated. This is best performed with a high-quality, high-power, microscope in the OR. At our center we have both a high-power lab scope in our operating room next to the surgeon and another in the adjacent full-time andrology lab for our andrologist to analyze the fluid.

Intraoperative Decision-Making: Perform a VV or VE?

One of the key points that separates out the true experts from many other doctors that perform reversals is the ability to review the vasal fluid intraoperatively and then, based on the microscopic findings, decide and perform a vasovasostomy or a vasoepididymostomy, whichever is indicated. This is perhaps the singularly most critical step that is so often overlooked by many doctors. There can never be a justifiable reason to not perform microscopic vasal fluid analysis.

Role of the Microscopic Fluid Analysis

The most important step to decide whether to perform a VV or a VE is the microscopic examination of the testicular vasal fluid. If sperm or parts are seen, then the testis-epididymis-vas system is patent, and therefore a VV is indicated. If no sperm or sperm parts are seen microscopically, which is consistent with deeper epididymal obstruction, then a VE is the correct procedure [16]. Look for the best sperm (longest tail length) when analyzing the vasal fluid. The number of sperm/cc or high-power field is estimated for whole, complete sperm, the % motile sperm, sperm with partial tails/cc, sperm heads, and sperm tails, or if no sperm, this is noted as well as if "snow" or degenerated parts are noted (Fig. 5.28). We have found that the presence of sperm with partial tails is a positive finding most often consistent with an open system and so the need for a VV. Despite the fact that many experts consider favorable gross findings with azoospermia a reason to perform a VV, we have not

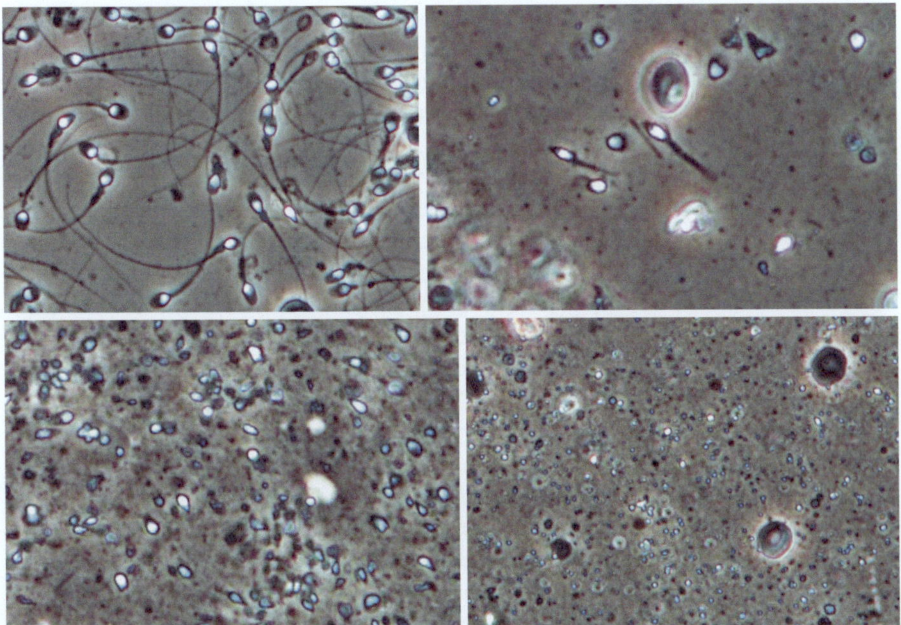

Fig. 5.28 Whole sperm, sperm with partial tails, sperm heads only, and "snow"-like debris. (Photo Credit: Sheldon Marks)

seen good results and so most often will proceed with a VE when no sperm are seen in the vasal fluid [16–28].

Here is our modification of the sperm grading system commonly used to categorize vasal sperm quality [29, 30].

Grade 1 – mainly normal, motile sperm
Grade 2 – mainly normal, nonmotile sperm
Grade 3 – sperm with partial tails
Grade 4 – mainly sperm heads
Grade 5 – only sperm heads
Grade 6 – no sperm

Indeterminate Vasal Fluid

When the vasal fluid is indeterminate and is not clearly consistent with an open system nor obvious deeper epididymal obstruction, then it is reasonable to take into account other fluid, patient, and partner factors to help with your decision-making re: whether to proceed with a vasovasostomy or move to perform a vasoepididymostomy. These include the gross fluid findings, the obstructive interval, the female partner's age, and reproductive timeline as well as the couple's preferences that you discussed with them in your conversations pre-reversal. In our practice with our high success rates with VEs, we believe that if we are not seeing sperm or parts as evidence of a non-obstructed system, then more often than not we will perform a vasoepididymostomy on that side.

We have found over the years that if the vasal fluid is indeterminate and we are uncertain if there is indeed deeper epididymal blockage, then when we proceed with the vasoepididymostomy and analyze the epididymal tubule fluid we are impressed with the good sperm count and motility. This reinforces the idea that the system was indeed obstructed, confirming that a vasoepididymostomy was the correct technique with indeterminate fluid. It is often reasonable to include in your decision-making the fluid findings and procedure performed on the contralateral side. For example, if one side has sperm and so a vasovasostomy is performed, then with indeterminate fluid on the other side we are more likely to default to a vasoepididy-mostomy. If both sides are indeterminate, then it may be reasonable to do a vasoepi-didymostomy on one side and then a vasovasostomy on the other, in an attempt to cover "all the bases" and give your patient the best chance for success. If the patient has a history of testosterone use, then one must consider that suppression may be the cause of azoospermia in the vasal fluid or it may be because of epididymal obstruction and make the best decision considering all the factors. This might be a good time to move to a diagnostic TESE to determine if there is normal, suppressed, or nonexistent spermatogenesis to help you in your decision-making.

Cross Contamination

It is important to be aware of and take precautions to prevent potential confounding cross contamination of sperm from one side to the other. This can be seen when sperm from the vasal or epididymal fluid on the first side are inadvertently introduced into the fluid or onto the glass slide to be analyzed from the contralateral vas. This would then falsely suggest that the second side's system is open with no deeper obstruction, and so a vasovasostomy may be incorrectly performed when in fact no sperm are present because of an epididymal blowout.

There are two scenarios where we have found this to be a potential problem.

1. If the tip of an instrument or of the Angiocath is used to stir the drop of vasal fluid from one side with the diluent before the slide is passed off, then sperm will be present on the tip. If that instrument or tip of the Angiocath is reused to also stir the fluid on the second side, it is possible that this may introduce rare sperm into otherwise sperm-free vasal fluid. These sperm would then be seen as evidence of system patency on that second side, and so you might incorrectly perform a vasovasostomy when a vasoepididymostomy is indicated.

2. The other possibility is that if an Angiocath is used to aspirate or flush one side which has sperm, then there may be some residual sperm up in the fluid within the end of the Angiocath, and this could then be accidentally introduced in vasal fluid from the second side, also leading to mistaken interpretation of the microscopic findings with sperm seen when there may be none, and so a vasovasostomy would be incorrectly performed.

To solve this potential problem, we now use two separate 3 cc syringes during surgery, each clearly labeled "Right" and "Left," for any irrigation or vasal barbotage. The left syringe can only be on the Mayo stand or used when working on the left side and is removed to the back table and the right syringe moved up when on the right side. We also only stir the vasal fluid on the glass slide with the tip of the Angiocath for that side and not the tip of any surgical instruments. This should eliminate any risks for cross contamination of sperm from one side to another.

Sperm Cryopreservation

At time of surgery, if the fluid is felt to be bankable in the three critical parameters of fluid volume, sperm count, and motility, and the patient has requested banking, then we aspirate the vasal fluid into a 1 cc TB syringe primed with HTF via a 24-gauge Angiocath and instill this into a sterile test tube with 0.5 cc of warmed HTF. When enough fluid has been aspirated from the vas, the test tube is then passed to the andrologist for analysis to determine if we have provided enough bankable sperm or if more fluid is needed. If acceptable, the specimen is processed for cryopreservation.

To Bank or Not to Bank

There is much debate about the usefulness and cost-effectiveness of banking sperm at the time of the vasectomy reversal [31–33]. Whether you address this with your patients or not, the patients are well aware of using banked sperm for in vitro fertilization with intracytoplasmic sperm injection (IVF + ICSI) from their friends and family as well as in the popular media. If you don't discuss the pros and cons of cryopreservation or make this option available for them, they may come back at a later date and wonder why this was not offered or performed. We believe that banking of sperm, when possible, provides a reasonable backup option for couples that may use this frozen sperm at some point in the future if the reversal is unsuccessful or if there are other health or fertility issues.

Sperm cryopreservation may be even more relevant at the time of a bilateral VE because of the lower success and more variable timeline for adequate sperm to appear in the ejaculate [34–37]. Of course, the added costs as well as the increased maternal and child health risks associated with IVF/ICSI should be discussed when counseling patients about the banking options and the use of frozen sperm [38, 39]. This then creates a new dilemma whether the anastomosis is the priority or the banking of sperm. If the patient requests sperm banking and you are performing a unilateral and especially a bilateral vasoepididymostomy, is it better to use a more caudal epididymal tubule which should theoretically allow for better sperm maturation and a technically easier anastomosis with no fluid banked or is it smarter to move up to a more cephalad tubule with increased chances to obtain bankable sperm for future IVF though with reduced likelihood for motile sperm in the ejaculate? Unless there is a short timeline for conception because of advanced maternal age, then the technical aspects of performing the best vasoepididymostomy should be the priority over the cryopreservation of sperm, though there are other experts that would argue that obtaining sperm for banking in this situation makes more sense because of the lower success and pregnancy after bilateral VEs.

References

1. American Urological Association; American Academy of Orthopaedic Surgeons. Antibiotic prophylaxis for urological patients with total joint replacements. J Urol. 2003;169:1796–7.
2. Wolf JS Jr, Bennett CJ, Dmochowski RR, Hollenbeck BK, Pearle MS, Schaeffer AJ. Best practice policy statement on urologic surgery antimicrobial prophylaxis. J Urol. 2008;179(4):1379–90.
3. Lowe G. Optimizing outcomes in vasectomy: how to ensure sterility and prevent complications. Transl Androl Urol. 2016;5(2):176–80.
4. Jarvi K, Grober ED, Lo KC, Patry G. Mini-incision microsurgical vasectomy reversal using no-scalpel vasectomy principles and instruments. Urology. 2008;72:913–5.
5. Grober ED, Jarvi K, Lo KC, Shin EJ. Mini-incision vasectomy reversal using no-scalpel vasectomy principles: efficacy and postoperative pain compared with traditional approaches to vasectomy reversal. Urology. 2011;77:602–6.
6. Werthman P. Mini-incision microsurgical vasoepididymostomy: a new surgical approach. Urology. 2007;70:794–6.
7. Schulster ML, Cohn MR, Najari BB, Goldstein M. Microsurgically assisted inguinal hernia repair and simultaneous male fertility procedures: rationale, technique and outcomes. J Urol. 2017;198(5):1168–74.
8. Schulster ML, Cohn MR, Najari BB, Goldstein M. Microsurgically assisted inguinal hernia repair and simultaneous male fertility procedures: rationale, technique and outcomes. J Urol. 2017;198(5):1168–74.
9. Nagler HM, Belletete BA, Gerber E, Dinlenc CZ. Laparoscopic retrieval of retroperitoneal vas deferens in vasovasostomy for postinguinal herniorrhaphy obstructive azoospermia. Fertil Steril. 2005;83:1842.
10. Shaeer OK, Shaeer KZ. Pelviscrotal vasovasostomy: refining and troubleshooting. J Urol. 2005;174:1935–7.
11. Lizza EF, Marmar JL, Schmidt SS, Lanasa JA Jr, Sharlip ID, Thomas AJ, Belker AM, Nagler HM. Transseptal crossed vasovasostomy. J Urol. 1985;134:1131–2.

12. Sabanegh E, Thomas AJ. Effectiveness of crossover transseptal vasoepididymostomy in treating complex obstructive azoospermia. Fertil Steril. 1995;63(2):392–5.
13. Crosnoe LE, Kim ED, Perkins AR, Marks MB, Burrows PJ, Marks SH. Angled vas cutter for vasovasostomy: technique and results. Fertil Steril. 2014;101(3):636–9.
14. Patel SR, Sigman M. Comparison of outcomes of vasovasostomy performed in the convoluted and straight vas deferens. J Urol. 2008;179:256–9.
15. Sandlow JI, Kolettis PN. Vasovasostomy in the convoluted vas deferens: indications and outcomes. J Urol. 2005;173:540–2.
16. Ostrowski KA, Tadros NN, Polackwich AS, McClure RD, Fuchs EF, Hedges JC. Factors and practice patterns that affect the decision for vasoepididymostomy. Can J Urol. 2017;24(1):8651–5.
17. Elzanaty S, Dohle GR. Vasovasostomy and predictors of vasal patency: a systematic review. Scand J Urol Nephrol. 2012;46:241–6.
18. Hinz S, Rais-Bahrami S, Weiske WH, Kempkensteffen C, Schrader M, Miller K, et al. Prognostic value of intraoperative parameters observed during vasectomy reversal for predicting postoperative vas patency and fertility. World J Urol. 2009;27(6):781–5.
19. Kirby EW, Hockenberry M, Lipshultz LI. Vasectomy reversal: decision making and technical innovations. Transl Androl Urol. 2017;6(4):753–60.
20. Kolettis PN, Burns JR, Nangia AK, Sandlow JI. Outcomes for vasovasostomy performed when only sperm parts are present in the vasal fluid. J Androl. 2006;27:565–7.
21. Kolettis PN, D'Amico AM, Box L, et al. Outcomes for vasovasostomy with bilateral intravasal azoospermia. J Androl. 2003;24:22–4.
22. Jarow JP, Sigman M, Buch JP, Oates RD. Delayed appearance of sperm after end-to-side vasoepididymostomy. J Urol. 1995;153:1156–8.
23. Ramasamy R, Mata DA, Jain L, Perkins AR, Marks SH, Lipshultz LI. Microscopic visualization of intravasal spermatozoa is positively associated with patency after bilateral microsurgical vasovasostomy. Andrology. 2015;3(3):532–5.
24. Scovell JM, Mata DA, Ramasamy R, Herrel LA, Hsiao W, Lipshultz LI. Association between the presence of sperm in the vasal fluid during vasectomy reversal and postoperative patency: a systematic review and meta-analysis. Urology. 2015;85(4):809–13.
25. Sheynkin YR, Chen ME, Goldstein M. Intravasal azoospermia: a surgical dilemma. BJU Int. 2000;85:1089–92.
26. Shin YS, Sang KSD, Park JK. Preoperative factors influencing postoperative results after vasovasostomy. World J Mens Health. 2012;30(3):177–82.
27. Sigman M. The relationship between intravasal sperm quality and patency rates after vasovasostomy. J Urol. 2004;171:307–9.
28. Smith RP, Khanna A, Kovac JR, et al. The significance of sperm heads and tails within the vasal fluid during vasectomy reversal. Indian J Urol. 2014;30:164–8.
29. Belker AM, Thomas AJ Jr, Fuchs EF, Konnak JW, Sharlip ID. Results of 1,469 microsurgical vasectomy reversals by the Vasovasostomy study group. J Urol. 1991;145:505–11.
30. Silber SJ. Microscopic vasectomy reversal. Fertil Steril. 1977;28:1191–202.
31. Glazier DB, Marmar JL, Mayer E, Gibbs M, Corson SL. The fate of cryopreserved sperm acquired during vasectomy reversals. J Urol. 1999;161:463–6.
32. Boyle KE, Thomas AJ Jr, Marmar JL, Hirshberg S, Belker AM, Jarow JP. Sperm harvesting and cryopreservation during vasectomy reversal is not cost effective. Fertil Steril. 2006;85:961–4.
33. Schrepferman CG, Carson MR, Sparks AE, Sandlow JI. Need for sperm retrieval and cryopreservation at vasectomy reversal. J Urol. 2001;166:1787–9.
34. Chan PT. The evolution and refinement of vasoepididymostomy techniques. Asian J Androl. 2013;15:49–55.
35. Peng J, Yuan Y, Zhang Z, Gao B, Song W, et al. Patency rates of microsurgical vasoepididymostomy for patients with idiopathic obstructive azoospermia: a prospective analysis of factors associated with patency – single-center experience. Urology. 2012;79:119–22.

36. Baker K, Sabanegh E. Obstructive azoospermia: reconstructive techniques and results. Clinics (Sao Paulo). 2013;68(Suppl 1):61–73.
37. Chan PT, Brandell RA, Goldstein M. Prospective analysis of outcomes after microsurgical intussusception vasoepididymostomy. BJU Int. 2005;96:598–601.
38. Pavlovich CP, Schlegel PN. Fertility options after vasectomy: a cost-effectiveness analysis. Fertil Steril. 1997;67(1):133–41.
39. Shridharani A, Sandlow JI. Vasectomy reversal versus IVF with sperm retrieval: which is better? Curr Opin Urol. 2010;20:503–9.

Chapter 6
Vasovasostomy: Multilayer Microsurgical Anastomosis

The specific technique that you use to perform a vasovasostomy is your own modification of techniques that have been developed and perfected over many decades by a handful of thought leaders in male reproductive microsurgery. Never satisfied with "good enough" or the status quo, these true leaders in our field have always been challenging themselves to develop new and improved techniques to improve the care and outcomes for all reversal patients. The following step-by-step techniques walk you through what we have found to work best for our patients, incorporating advances by so many. Every time I perform a reversal, I marvel at how far we have come and wonder what the newest advances will be.

Evolution of Vasovasostomy Techniques

The techniques for the modern microsurgical vasovasostomy have evolved with advances and refinements from the modified one-layer to the two-layer to the current multilayer reversal [1–4]. The technique that you choose to use to perform vasectomy reversals is usually a variation of the technique that you learned during residency or fellowship [5].

Of course, the patient's anatomy and post-vasectomy changes may necessitate modifications and changes to another technique. Concerns over your skills, time, and costs can play a role in deciding what technique you will do and what is best for that patient.

I did ask one leading educator in this day and age where most experts agree that performing the multilayer anastomosis provides the highest success, why he still taught the less precise modified one-layer. He explained that he knew that his residents would only perform a rare reversal, maybe a few a year at best, and so would not have been able to perfect the skills to perform a more challenging multilayer

© Springer Nature Switzerland AG 2019
S. H. F. Marks, *Vasectomy Reversal*,
https://doi.org/10.1007/978-3-030-00455-2_6

closure. He went on to explain that he taught them the modified one-layer technique because it would still provide good results, even with less experienced hands. There are some leaders in the vasectomy reversal world that use the modified one-layer technique because it is easier and faster to perform, with what they believe to be good results. Another expert explained that he felt that it was important to use this technique to ensure that all suture knots are outside of the vas.

Each technique offers advantages and disadvantages to the patient and the surgeon. Some are faster or easier or use less sutures and so are less expensive to perform. But I would caution that if patients understand their options, they will rarely want the technique that is faster or easier for the surgeon. They are spending a lot of money investing in their dream and expect the absolute very highest chances for success. All of the techniques described will be microsurgical. The modified one-layer is the easiest to perform, takes less time, and is believed to use less sutures so is thought to be less expensive, with good results in experienced hands. The formal two-layer is technically more challenging and so requires more skills to precisely anastomose the mucosal layers and then the muscularis layers. The multilayer (three to four layers) closure, which is more anatomically precise, what I prefer, and the technique used by most top experts provides the highest level of success though, as with the two-layer, is technically more demanding. Costs for the multilayer vasovasostomy can be drastically reduced to three suture packets per case utilizing modifications described in the step-by-step instructions below. This cost-effective modification allows for the multilayer repair to actually use less microsutures than the modified one-layer closure.

Microdots

Microdots are very helpful in maintaining orientation of the vas and allowing for more precise and consistent placement of the microsutures [6, 7]. The most difficult aspect to placing microdots is finding a true microtipped marker, with consistency in production and quality control. Most often we have found that even with the same product from the same manufacturer and vendor, the tip can vary widely in how fine the tip really is and presence of significant irregularities. Sometimes the tip is very sharp and ideal, while other times it may be blunt or splayed apart creating more of a paw print rather than a fine microdot. Before placing the microdots, dry the face of the vas with a dab of an eye spear.

I usually place six dots equidistant, starting at 12 o'clock position, at the junction two-thirds in from the outer vas and one-third in from the lumen. For those that prefer seven or eight mucosal sutures, then place that number of microdots. With the improvement with the angled vas cutting forceps, we modified the microdot technique to place double dots at the 12 o'clock position to maintain orientation (Fig. 6.1). In addition to the microdots, we highlight the circumference of the mucosal edge with the micropen to better visualize of the edge of the lumen.

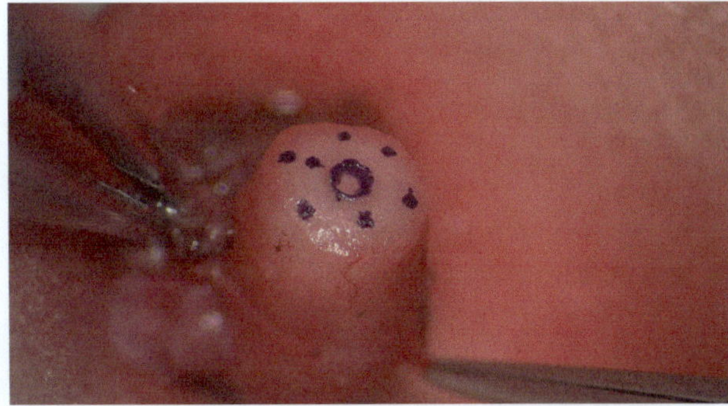

Fig. 6.1 Microdots to allow for precise placement of the microsutures with a double dot at the 12 o'clock position to maintain orientation. (Photo Credit: Sheldon Marks)

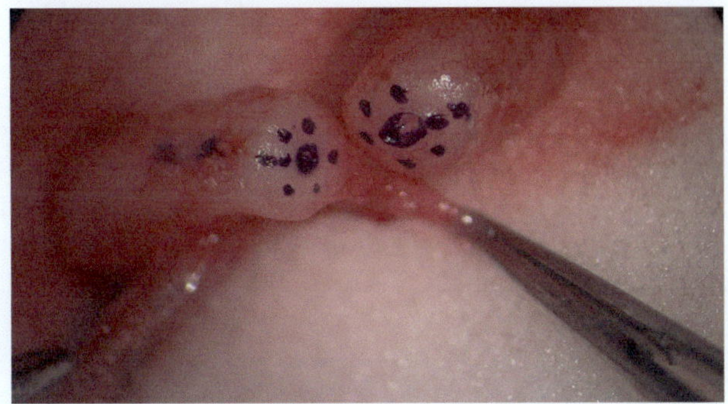

Fig. 6.2 The transected ends of the vas should be secured adjacent to each other. (Photo Credit: Sheldon Marks)

Techniques to Stabilize the Vas

In order to make performing the anastomosis easy, the transected vasal ends should be secured to bring the ends adjacent to each other, off tension, for the placement of the microsutures. This is often referred to as "kissing lumens" (Fig. 6.2). Senior reversal experts will tell you that quite often the most difficult aspect of any reversal can be the setup. Finding and bringing together the ends of the vas or vas to the correct epididymal tubule is a challenge and sometimes the most time-consuming aspect of a reversal. There are three common ways most experts secure the transected ends of the vas adjacent to each other on a stable platform.

1. Goldstein vas approximating clamp
2. Microwipe technique
3. Stay sutures

Goldstein Vas Approximating Clamp

The articulated Goldstein MicrospikeTM approximator clamp (ASSI.MSPK3678) secures both ends of the vas with tiny microspikes, which secure the vas in place allowing for stable vasal anastomosis [8]. The four variations of the Goldstein clamp

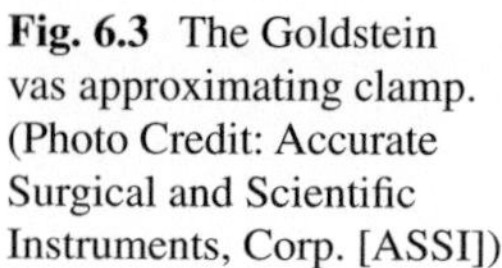

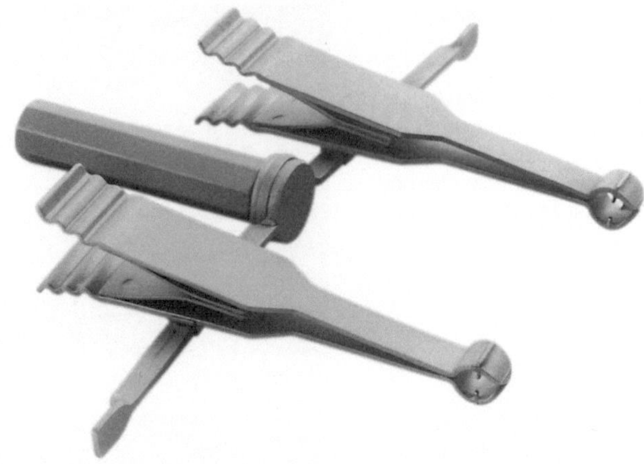

Fig. 6.3 The Goldstein vas approximating clamp. (Photo Credit: Accurate Surgical and Scientific Instruments, Corp. [ASSI])

allow for the repair to be easily rotated 90–180° as needed to place additional sutures. This clamp is very popular and perhaps the most common technique used. In the past, some have commented that there have been issues with the microspikes and sutures being caught in the device with breaking of the suture or the needle inadvertently popping off (Fig. 6.3).

Surgical Microwipe Technique

This approach, which we developed decades ago, is what I prefer to use to secure both ends of the vas together during the repair. This technique provides several advantages over the other techniques.

1. Very inexpensive, easy to use instrument Microwipe (Ivalon by Fabco, 2 mm 8.25 cm × 8.25 cm).
2. Provides a white background, which allows for better visualization of the microneedle and suture. As we all know, these can be difficult to see on regular blue drapes or in the tissues.
3. If a microneedle should pop off, then you know it is not in the wound.
4. The tissue wipe also covers and protects the underlying tissues, keeping them moist. The only tissues seen are the ends of the vas protruding through small holes.
5. This technique provides a stable platform that also allows you to rotate the vas as needed. When the anastomosis is completed on that side, it is simply cut away. The underlying peri-vasal tissues are then re-examined under the microscope, looking for any bleeding sites that need to be addressed.

The modified Microwipe is easy to make before or at the time of the reversal. Two small 3 × 3.75 cm pieces are cut from the larger surgical 7.5 × 7.5 cm surgical wipe. Two 1 to 2 mm defects are created in each piece of a moistened Microwipe.

To do this the surgical wipe is folded in half and then in half again, and a tip of the corner is excised, leaving a small defect in the wipe (Fig. 6.4). The peri-vasal adventitia at the end of the transected vas is grabbed by the tip of a microhemostat and pulled though the defect. Once 1 or 2 cm of the vasal end is brought through each hole, the vas is secured by clamping the adventitia to the edge of the Microwipe defect. This can be secured with one or two microhemostats for each segment of the vas, above or below the wipe (Fig. 6.5).

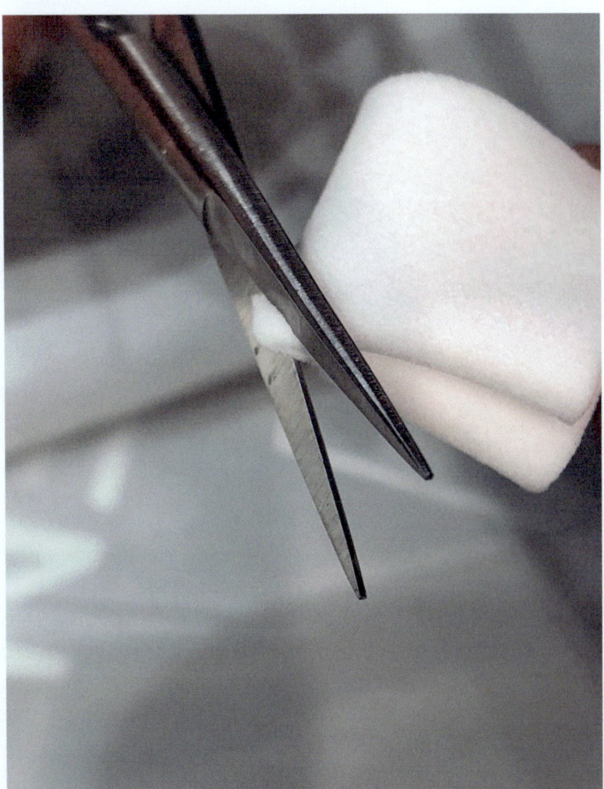

Fig. 6.4 Creating the defects in the Microwipe. (Photo Credit: Sheldon Marks)

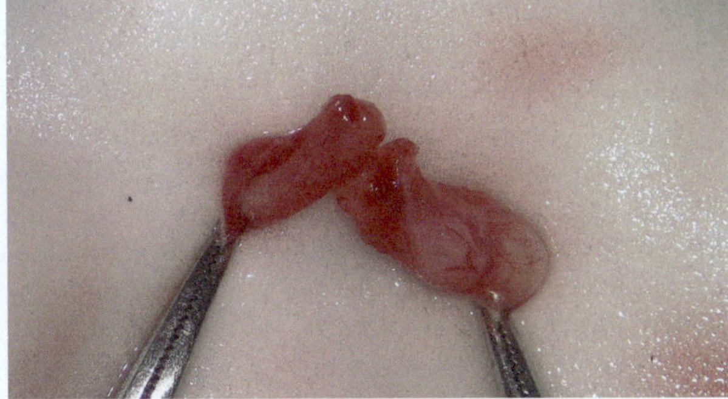

Fig. 6.5 The ends of the vas are brought through the defects in the Microwipe and secured with a microhemostat to the peri-vasal adventitia. (Photo Credit: Sheldon Marks)

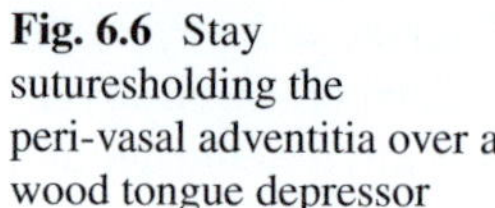

Fig. 6.6 Stay suturesholding the peri-vasal adventitia over a wood tongue depressor

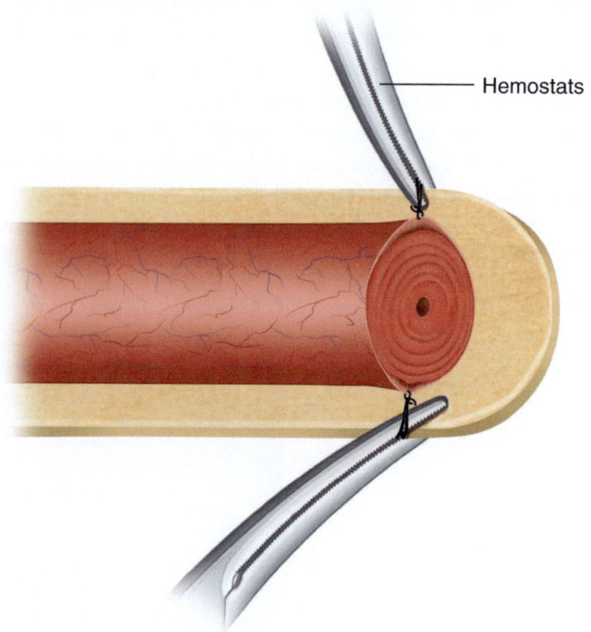

Stay Suture Technique

The stay suture technique to secure the vas requires placement of stay sutures, usually of a heavier suture, secured in the peri-vasal adventitia of the ends of the vas. These stay sutures are then tied together or secured to each other with microhemostats, which can be secured to or over a sterile wooden tongue depressor, to draw the ends of the vas together, off tension. Some use a portion of or one finger of a sterile glove over the tongue blade to provide a protective backdrop for the anastomosis (Fig. 6.6).

Rotate the Vas

Whichever of these or other vasal stabilization methods or techniques you use, it is important to be able to easily rotate the posterior vas anteriorly to better visualize and address suture placement. One approach when completed with the posterior sutures is to rotate the vas a complete 180° to bring the posterior tissues up anteriorly and expose the tissues that need to be approximated. Then place and tie the sutures, starting laterally, working toward the midline. The other technique to see the posterior layers is to rotate the vas only 90°, address the tissues you can see, and then rotate the vas back 180° the other way to address the opposite side. The method you use may be the same or may vary from patient to patient and will depend on the patients' anatomy, your preferences, as well as the amount of vasal length and flexibility.

The Cost-Effective Multilayer Vasovasostomy

This is the technique I have developed over the past decades and many thousands of reversals and use daily for a very cost-effective multilayer vasovasostomy. As addressed earlier, this is what works best for me and provides consistently very high success. Throughout your own practice, you will develop your own technique that works best for you. I hope that included here are some insights, tips, and pearls that you may find useful to incorporate into your own technique, in combination with insights and suggestions from other experts you will pick up throughout your practice.

This cost-effective technique uses only a total of 3 microsuture packets for both sides of a bilateral vasovasostomy without compromised quality or outcomes as compared to the 15–20 sutures for a standard multilayer VV. I use a single packet of a long 6 inch 10-0 nylon double-armed suture (Sharpoint $_{TM}$ 10-0 AA-2334) for all sutures of the mucosal layers on both sides. We cut the long suture in half yielding two separate 10-0 sutures each (Fig. 6.7) with 3 inches of suture on a 100 micron needle, which is usually plenty of length for the six or seven mucosal stitches we place on a side. Then we use a single 9-0 nylon 5 inch (Sharpoint $_{TM}$ 9-0 AA-1825) for the muscularis sutures on both sides and one 7-0 nylon suture (Ethilon $_{TM}$ 7-0 18 inch/45 cm black nylon monofilament) for the adventitial layer stitches. Of course, if suture costs are no concern, then you can use a short 2.5 inch double- armed 10-0 (Sharpoint $_{TM}$ 10-0 AA-2492) for each mucosal suture placed.

The standard vasovasostomy technique that has been taught over the years is to use an individual double-armed 2.5 inch 10-0 suture for each of the six to eight inner layer mucosal sutures [9, 10]. The needles are passed from the mucosal layer in-to-out of the inner muscularis on both the abdominal and testicular vas (Fig. 6.8). This then requires a separate double-armed suture for each stitch thrown which can add

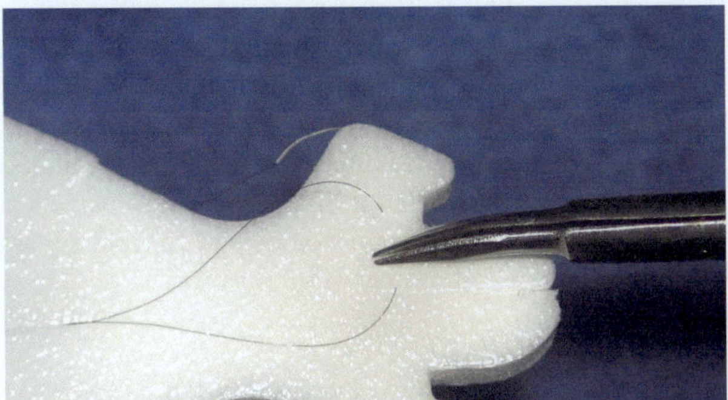

Fig. 6.7 Dividing the long 6 inch 10-0 nylon double-armed suture to create two 3 inch 10-0 nylon single-armed sutures. (Photo Credit: Sheldon Marks)

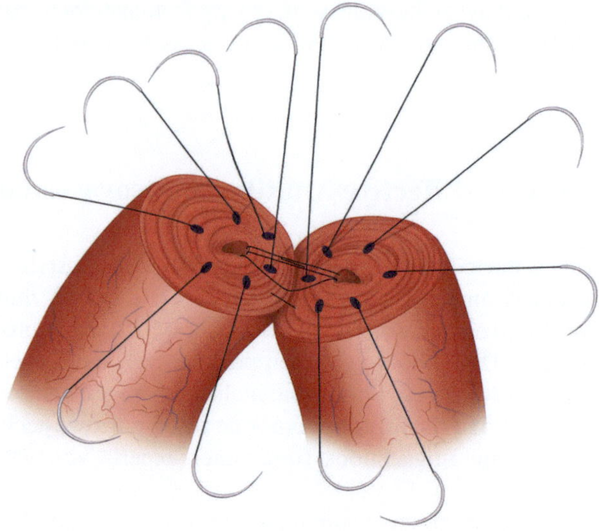

Fig. 6.8 Standard technique with an individual 2.5 inch double-armed 10-0 needle placed in to out for each of the six to eight stitches on both the abdominal and testicular lumens

up to 6–8 sutures per side, for a total of 12–16 just for the mucosal sutures. Then add to this one 9-0 suture for the muscularis on each side and an additional 7-0 suture for the adventitial layers, and this technique requires a total of 15–19 microsutures, at approximately $50 a suture for a cost of $750–$950 or more per vasovasostomy as compared to our cost-effective technique of 3 sutures total with a cost of only $150 per VV [10, 11].

Placing the Vasovasostomy Sutures, Layer by Layer

There are two approaches that most experts use to place the initial posterior microsutures. One is to place three interrupted posterior muscularis sutures to bring the two transected faces of the vas together and then the posterior mucosal and then anterior mucosal sutures [12]. The other technique, which I prefer most often, is to place the posterior 10-0 mucosal sutures first and then the anterior mucosa and then the muscularis sutures. If there are concerns that the anastomosis might be on any tension, then I use the "muscularis first" approach to secure the vasal ends adjacent to each other before placing the posterior mucosal sutures. More often than not, however, I find it technically easier to complete the mucosal lumen anastomosis first before addressing the muscularis sutures. Whether placing the mucosal or muscularis sutures, we have found that it is very helpful to place a cellulose foam surgical spear (ASSI 53810) behind the anastomosis to lift and separate the vas, providing better exposure of the vasal lumens (Fig. 6.9).

Fig. 6.9 Foam surgical spear placed behind the anastomosis to gently lift and separate the vas and provide better visualization of the edges of the luminal mucosa. (Photo Credit: Sheldon Marks)

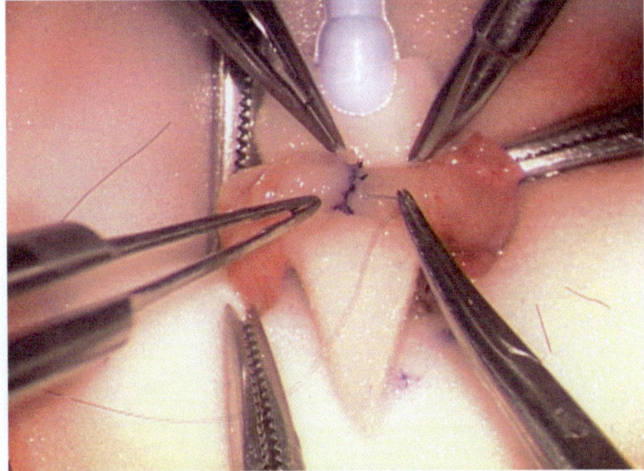

Fig. 6.10 Mucosal 10-0 nylon sutures placed at the 4, 6, and 8 o'clock position. (Photo Credit: Sheldon Marks)

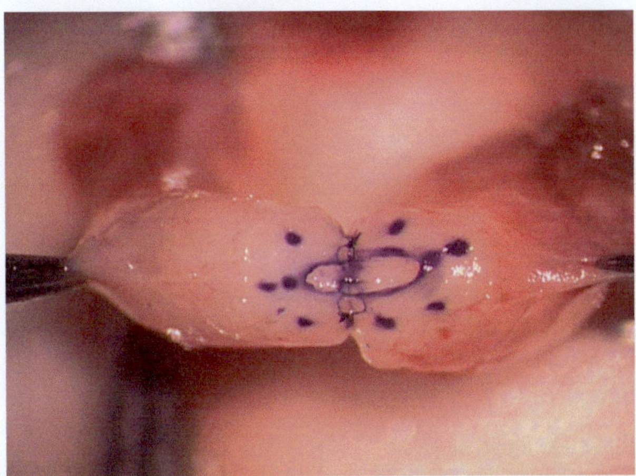

Inner Mucosal Layer Before Posterior Muscularis Technique

First place the 10-0 nylon suture on a 70 micron needle at the 6 o'clock position of the vasal lumen mucosa, always out-to-in on the testicular vas and then in-to-out on the abdominal vas, and tie. Then repeat placing sutures at the 8 o'clock and 4 o'clock position (Fig. 6.10). The sutures should include 1 to 2 mm of the mucosa inside the lumen edge and exit at about one-third of the muscularis (Fig. 6.11). Then irrigate and place but do not tie the 10, 2, and finally the 12 o'clock position sutures (Fig. 6.12). Re-examine the sutures and lumens to confirm that the sutures have not inadvertently included the back wall of the mucosa or are intertwined with another

Fig. 6.11 Sutures to include about one-third of the inner muscularis

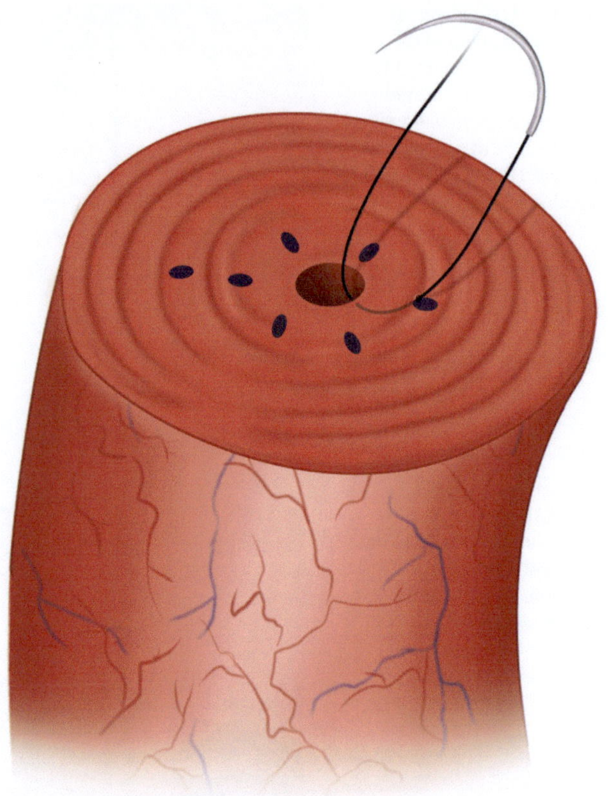

Fig. 6.12 Final mucosal sutures placed but not tied at the 10, 12, and 2 o'clock position. (Photo Credit: Sheldon Marks)

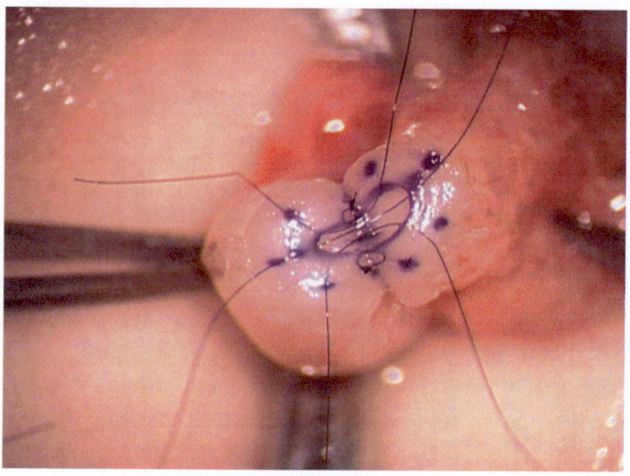

suture. Then tie the 10 and then 2, and lastly irrigate the lumen and tie the 12 o'clock sutures (Fig. 6.13).

Middle Muscularis Layer

When all of the inner layer mucosal sutures are placed and tied, then place and tie through the outer one-third of the muscularis each interrupted 9-0 nylon on a 100 micron one-half circle cutting needle circumferentially at 1 mm equidistant intervals. Start at the 12 o'clock position, and then proceed around the vas, placing and tying each suture out-to-in and then in-to-out (Fig. 6.14). Then when you have gone as far as you can easily, go back to the 12 o'clock suture, and begin placing sutures as you roll the vas to expose the remaining unapproximated muscularis. It may be easier to rotate the vas 90° in both directions or 180° to easily visualize and place the muscularis sutures. As with all previous sutures, it is important to irrigate with a pulse of LR or NS just before tying down the first knot to remove any debris, residual sperm, or blood clots. Be careful to not transect the inner mucosal sutures with the tip of the 9-0 needle.

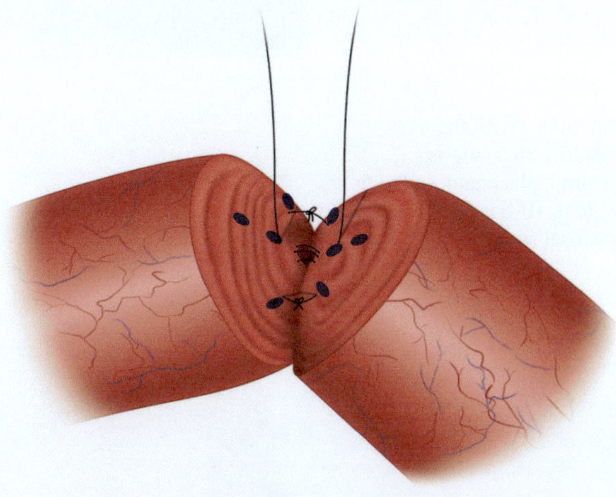

Fig. 6.13 Tie both of the lateral mucosal sutures and then the 12 o'clock suture

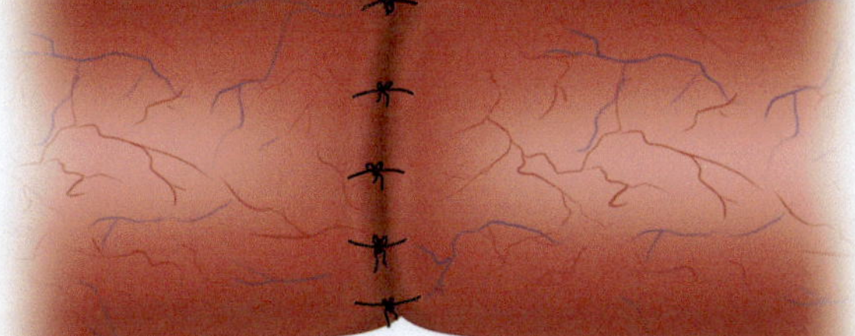

Fig. 6.14 Interrupted 9-0 nylon muscularis sutures to include about one-third of the outermost muscularis tissues, tied as they are placed circumferentially

Placing the Posterior Muscularis Before Posterior Mucosa Technique

Using same techniques as described, start with the 6 o'clock posterior vas muscularis 9–0 suture and tie, and then place and tie the 8 and 4 o'clock position 9-0 sutures. (Fig. 6.15). Then position the foam eye spear to better visualize the posterior lumen mucosa, and place and tie the 6 o'clock 10-0 nylon, (Fig. 6.16), followed by the 8 and 4 o'clock position mucosal 10-0 sutures. (Fig. 6.17).

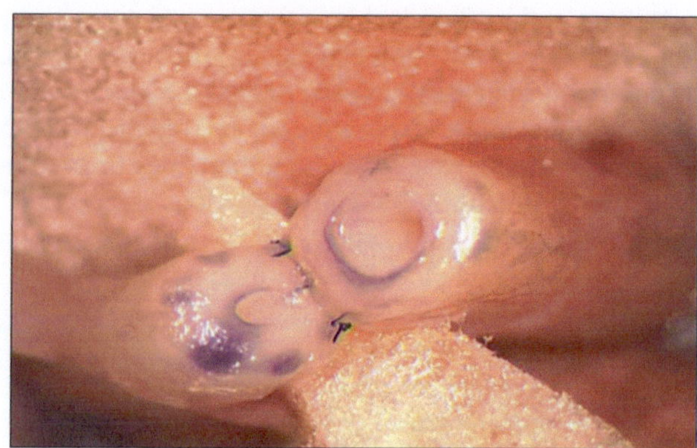

Fig. 6.15 First place and tie the 6 o'clock and then the 8 and 4 o'clock position 9-0 nylon sutures

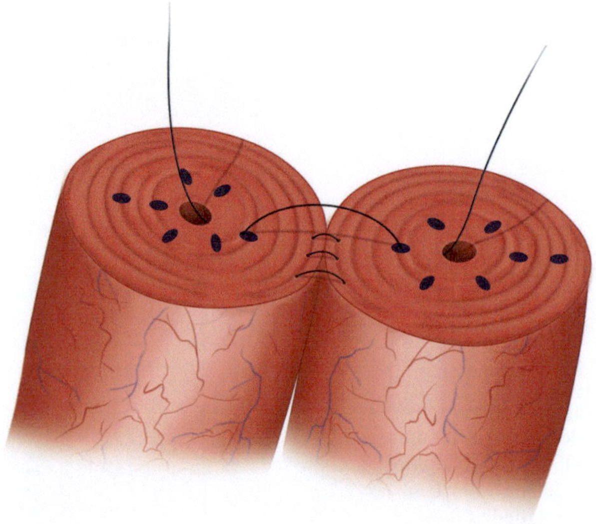

Fig. 6.16 With the posterior muscularis secured, place and tie the 6 o'clock 10-0 nylon mucosal suture

Fig. 6.17 Place and tie
the 8 and 4 o'clock
position mucosal 10-0
sutures

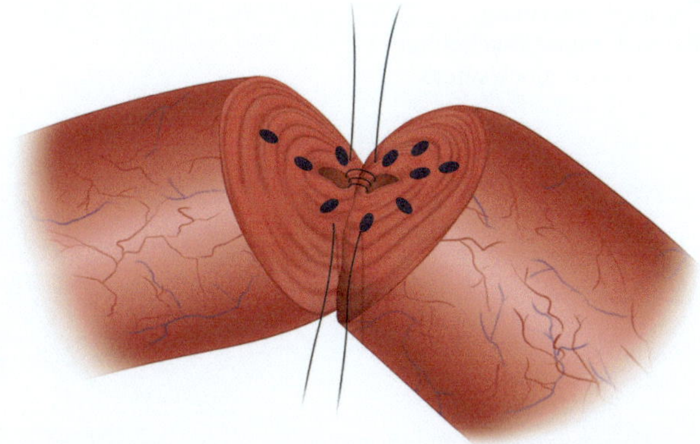

Fig. 6.18 Place but do not
tie the 10, 2, and finally the
12 o'clock position
mucosal 10-0 nylon
sutures. (Photo Credit:
Sheldon Marks)

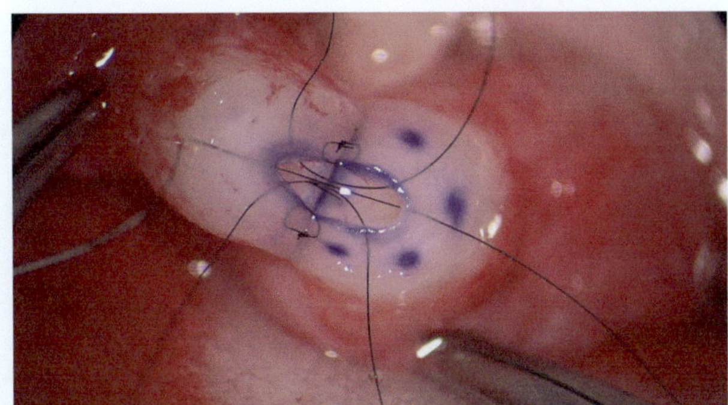

Anterior Mucosal Sutures

Then as with the previous technique, irrigate the lumen, and place but do not tie the 10, 2, and finally the 12 o'clock position 10-0 nylon sutures, allowing for visualization of the mucosal edges (Fig. 6.18). Re-examine the sutures and luminal mucosa to confirm that the sutures have not inadvertently included the back wall of the mucosa or are intertwined with another suture. Then tie the 10 o'clock and then 2 o'clock and lastly a final irrigation of the lumen and tie the 12 o'clock 10-0 sutures (Fig. 6.19).

Anterior Muscularis

As described above, place and tie the remaining interrupted muscularis 9-0 nylon sutures each 1 mm apart completing the layer (Fig. 6.20).

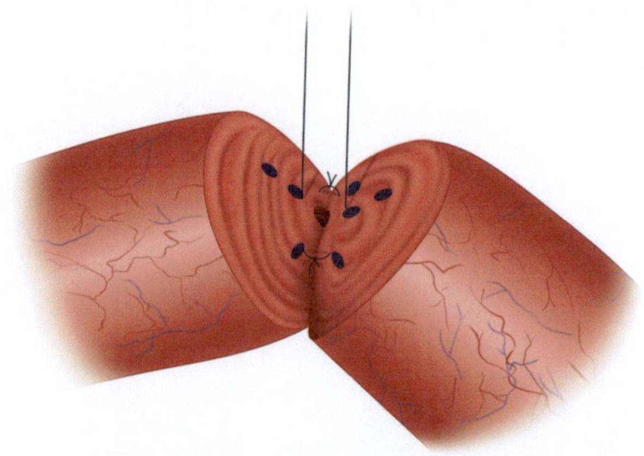

Fig. 6.19 Tie lateral mucosal sutures first before the final 12 o'clock suture

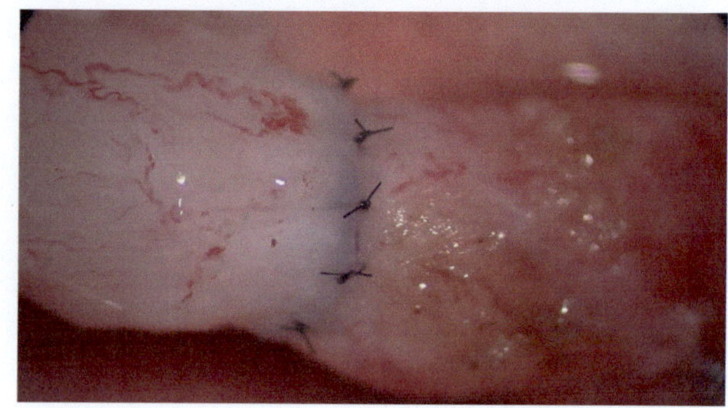

Fig. 6.20 Place and tie the remaining interrupted muscularis 9-0 nylon sutures. (Photo Credit: Sheldon Marks)

Peri–vasal Adventitial Layer(s)

The adventitia is then approximated with interrupted 7-0 nylon sutures to draw the edges together, prevent any tension on the underlying anastomosis, and provide a healthy blood supply to the repair. Depending on the diameter of the vas and how much adventitial tissue is available, this might require anywhere from 6 to 12 sutures, in 1 or 2 layers (Fig. 6.21). This is also the time to tie off any remaining small peri-vasal blood vessels. Once the vasovasostomy on the first side is completed, then re-examine through the microscope for any bleeding, and replace the vas back into the hemiscrotum. Then repeat these steps on the contralateral side.

Closing

When both sides are completed, we reinfiltrate the subcutaneous tissues with local anesthetic and then reinspect for any bleeding that may have started up and address if identified. The layers are closed with interrupted 4-0 Vicryl and the skin

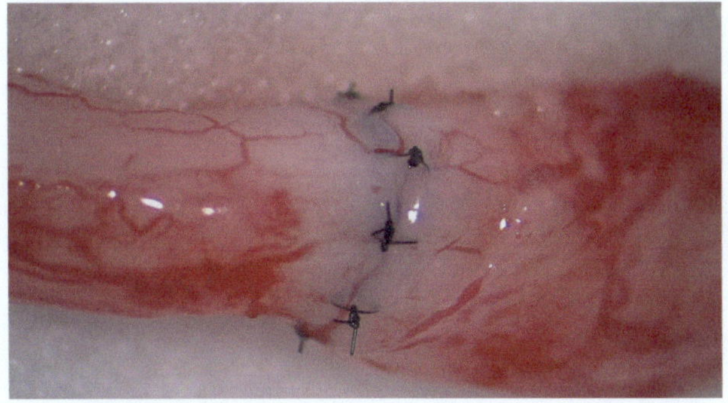

Fig. 6.21 Finally approximate the outer adventitial tissues in one to two layers with interrupted 7-0 nylon sutures. (Photo Credit: Sheldon Marks)

approximated with a 5-0 running monofilament absorbable (Monocryl$_{TM}$, Caprosyn$_{TM}$, or equivalent) subcuticular stitch. Then apply bacitracin ointment and hold pressure on the incision for 5 min, redress the patient, and place an athletic supporter with ice after arrival in recovery.

Modified One-Layer Vasovasostomy

This technique is the one most commonly used by general urologists as this is considered to be technically easier and faster to perform with less sutures used. The modified one-layer does not require the level of microsurgical skills necessary for a precise multilayer vasovasostomy. Not only is the modified one-layer reversal easier to perform; many believe that in this age of cost control, since it uses less sutures, the reversal can be performed at less expense for the patient and the center. They do acknowledge that the success rates, though not as high as with a formal multilayer closure, are considered to be "good enough." It is the author's opinion that any cost justification for performing the modified one-layer technique with a success of 90% is negated by using the "cost-conscious" microsurgical multilayer vasovasostomy as described above, which actually uses less microsutures than the modified one-layer but with higher success at 99.5%.

Technique for Modified One-Layer Vasovasostomy

The vasal prep, transection, and securing of the vas with fluid interpretation are the same as described with the multilayer VV. The bottom line is that instead of multiple sutures placed for each layer, the modified one-layer technique uses four full-thickness sutures followed by four or more muscularis sutures.

Once the two ends of the vas are secured adjacent to each other as described above, a 9-0 nylon double-armed suture is placed in-to-out full thickness from the mucosal layer out through the muscularis (Fig. 6.22) starting at the 6 o'clock

Fig. 6.22 Modified one-layer vasovasostomy. The first 9-0 nylon double-armed suture is placed in-to-out full thickness from the mucosal layer out through the muscularis starting at the 6 o'clock position on both the abdominal and testicular vas

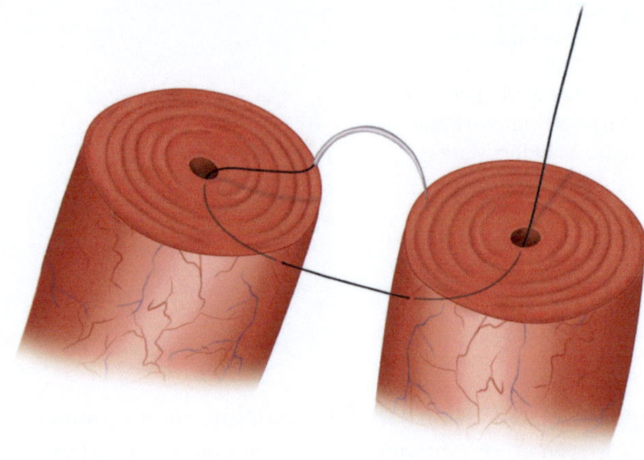

Fig. 6.23 Three additional full-thickness sutures are similarly placed at the 3, the 9, and then the 12 o'clock position

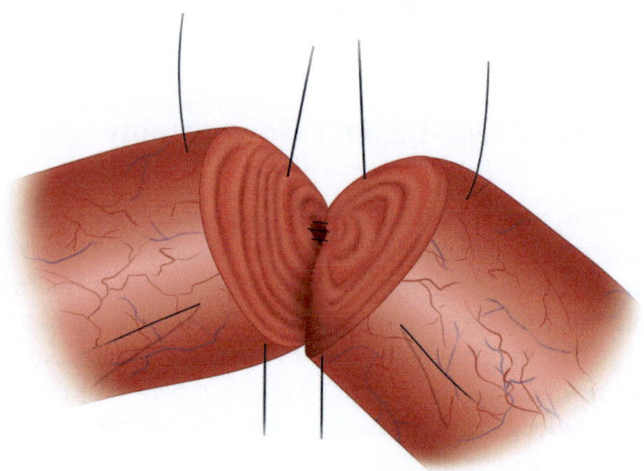

position on both the abdominal and testicular vas and then tied. Then additional full-thickness sutures are similarly placed at the 3 o'clock and then 9 o'clock position of both ends but not tied. The lumen is flushed, and the final suture is placed full thickness at the 12 o'clock position out both the abdominal and testicular vas (Fig. 6.23). Then the three sutures are tied, starting laterally and finally with the 12 o'clock suture.

Then four interrupted 7-0 nylon sutures are then placed in the outer one-third of the vasal muscularis, positioned equidistant in between the tied full-thickness sutures (Fig. 6.24). Additional 7-0 nylon sutures can be placed as needed in the muscularis. Care must be taken to not inadvertently cut the full-thickness suture with the point of the needle on the 7-0 nylon when passing the suture.

Fig. 6.24 Four interrupted 7-0 nylon sutures are then placed in the outer one-third of the vasal muscularis, positioned equidistant in between the tied full-thickness sutures

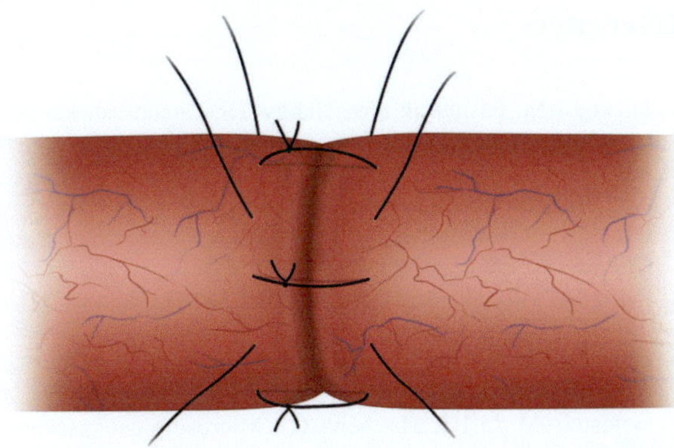

Fig. 6.25 Two-layer vasovasostomy with inner mucosal layer approximated with interrupted 10-0 nylon and the outer muscularis layer with 9-0 nylon sutures

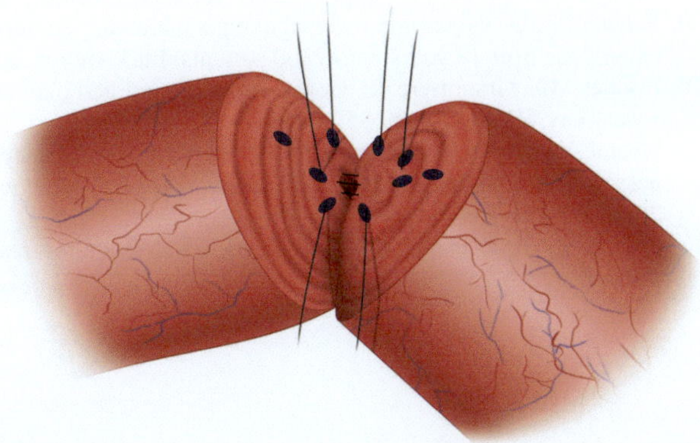

Two-Layer Vasovasostomy

The two-layer vasovasostomy technique evolved as a result of the desire for a more precise closer with a higher success than the modified one-layer. The anastomosis of both layers requires specific and rapidly perishable microsurgical skills and requires more time. The two-layer approach uses the same first steps as a multilayer repair except that you perform only the mucosal and then the muscularis layers without the approximation of the outermost adventitial layers (Fig. 6.25). My own thoughts are if you are going to go the trouble to perfect and fine-tune your micro-surgical skills to address the challenges and nuances of performing a precise muco-sal and then muscularis closure, you might as well approximate the outer adventitial layer or layers with several 7-0 nylon sutures to reduce any risks for tension on the repair and to replace the fat and vascular supply over the underlying anastomosis.

References

1. Dickey RM, Pastuszak AW, Hakky TS, Chandrashekar A, Ramasamy R, Lipshultz LI. The evolution of vasectomy reversal. Curr Urol Rep. 2015 Jun;16(6):40.
2. Kim HH, Goldstein M. History of vasectomy reversal. Urol Clin North Am. 2009 Aug;36(3):359–73.
3. Baker K, Sabaneugh E Jr. Obstructive azoospermia: reconstructive techniques and results. Clinics. 2013;68(Suppl1):61–73.
4. Pastuszak AW, Wenker EP, Lipshultz LI. The history of microsurgery in urology. Urology. 2015;85(5):971–4.
5. Crain DS, Roberts JL, Amling CL. Practice patterns in vasectomy reversal surgery: results of a questionnaire study among practicing urologists. J Urol. 2004;171:311–5.
6. Goldstein M, Li PS, Matthews GJ. Microsurgical vasovasostomy: the microdot technique of precision suture placement. J Urol. 1998;159:188–90.
7. Walsh PC, editor. Campbell's urology. 8th ed. Philadelphia: WB Saunders; 2002. p. 1533–87.
8. Goldstein M. Microspike approximator for vasovasostomy. J Urol. 1985;134:74.
9. Schwarzer JU. Vasectomy reversal using a microsurgical three-layer technique: one surgeon's experience over 18 years with 1300 patients. Int J Androl. 2012;35:706–13.
10. Fischer MA, Grantmyre JE. Comparison of modified one- and two-layer microsurgical vasovasostomy. BJU Int. 2000;85:1085–8.
11. Nyame YA, Babbar P, Almassi N, Polackwich AS, Sabanegh E. Comparative cost-effectiveness analysis of modified 1-layer versus formal 2-layer vasovasostomy technique. J Urol. 2016;195:434–8.
12. Ramasamy R, Schlegel PN. Vasectomy and vasectomy reversal: an update. Indian J Urol. 2011;27(1):92–7.

Chapter 7
Vasoepididymostomy: End-to-Side Longitudinal Multilayer Intussusception

A microsurgical multilayer vasoepididymostomy is considered one of the most technically challenging microsurgical procedures in medicine and requires highly refined microsurgical skills to achieve good results. These skills are difficult to learn, take regular practice to perfect, and are rapidly perishable, so performing a VE is not for the "occasional" microsurgeon [1, 2]. The modern multilayer vasoepididymostomy has evolved over the past decades from an end-to-end connection to the standard end-to-side five- to six-suture approach to the three-suture horizontal intussusception to the current longitudinal two-suture intussusception multilayer technique [3]. Advances in techniques, microsutures, and microneedles yielding the highest success make the current end-to-side intussusception anastomosis the most preferred approach by most top reversal experts.

Indications for a Vasoepididymostomy

A vasoepididymostomy is the technique that should be performed, independent of the obstructive interval, when the gross and microscopic analysis of the vasal fluid shows findings such as no sperm, old, degenerated sperm heads or only "snow-like" debris. This absence of sperm or sperm parts is consistent with a deeper, epididymal tubule blowout with obstruction, blocking the flow of sperm into the vas. The technique you choose for a vasoepididymostomy will depend on the surgeon's skills and experience as well as the post-vasectomy anatomy and the size of the epididymal tubule. Though most often an end-to-side longitudinal two-suture vasoepididymostomy is indicated, if the epididymal tubulotomy is lengthy, then the standard five- or six-suture end-to-side technique may be more appropriate.

© Springer Nature Switzerland AG 2019
S. H. F. Marks, *Vasectomy Reversal*,
https://doi.org/10.1007/978-3-030-00455-2_7

Vasoepididymostomy Success

In experienced hands, you can expect to achieve a 70–90% success for a vasoepididymostomy, though with a more variable and unpredictable return of sperm to ejaculate. Though there are many variables that impact on success, the patency after a VE is directly dependent on the skills and experience of the microsurgeon [4–9]. Though we do the same technique, the same way, day after day over many years, we have found that there is no way to accurately predict whether sperm will be seen right away with the first post-reversal semen analysis or delayed a few months or even up to 12–18 months or more. Many top experts believe that if you cannot perform a VE regularly with good results, then it is not in the patient's best interests to even start a reversal as the chances are good even with a short obstructive interval that you may need to perform a bypass.

Vasoepididymostomy: Step by Step

As with the vasovasostomy, these are the steps and techniques we have found to be effective when performing a microsurgical vasoepididymostomy at our center. You are encouraged to think about your own techniques and consider what we describe to see if there are any tips or pointers that you might want to incorporate into your own practice.

Examining the Epididymis

After the testicle is delivered and the tunica vaginalis opened, examine and palpate the testicle, noting the size, consistency, and orientation or if there are any irregularities, adhesions, or scarring. This is important to be sure there are no testicular masses or areas of induration that might represent an unsuspected malignancy. Next examine the epididymis, looking for any findings that might localize the region of the epididymal blowout and obstruction to include any areas of discoloration (brown, black, or yellow) or palpable induration. Look for dilated tubules as well as the color of the fluid within the tubules. Intratubular fluid can be clear, murky, or shades of white, yellow, or brown and often changes along the length of the epididymis. You will often see dilated tubules filled with white fluid below the blockage. You will also identify any adhesions, epididymal cysts, or scarring that may pose additional challenges to performing the vasoepididymostomy.

Identifying the Target Epididymal Tubule

There is no clear, definitive guidance on how to select the right epididymal tubule when performing a vasoepididymostomy that is agreed upon by most reversal experts. Several years ago, I asked a panel of leading reversal doctors what tubule fluid factors they each used to decide if a tubule was acceptable or not. Every respected expert had a different idea as to what they believed to be the most important factors to use. What aspects of epididymal fluid make the tubule ideal for the anastomosis? Many experts tell me that they look for sperm as evidence of patency or even sperm with partial tails. Others prefer to see motile sperm in the epididymal fluid before they will perform the vasoepididymostomy. Some want to see sperm or sperm with partial tails with good epididymal fluid volume. I am always amazed that there are surprisingly few papers on the subject. These are my thoughts, based on thousands of reversals over many decades, as well as input from other experts so that you can decide on your own how to select a tubule. Deciding which tubule to use is still one of those topics where you need to base your decisions on your own "lessons learned" experience performing vasoepididymostomies as well as expert opinion from our colleagues.

What Is the Ideal Target Tubule for Vasoepididymostomy?

At our reversal center, we use a number of factors to describe the ideal epididymal tubule that we will select for a vasoepididymostomy. Often selecting which is the best epididymal tubule to use comes with years of trial-and-error experience. Even then, many times we discover that the tubule that we thought was ideal was found to have no sperm, and so we are forced to find and prep one or more tubules a few mm up the epididymis until we find one with acceptable fluid and usable physical characteristics.

Six Factors to Use to Select a Tubule

At our center, the ideal epididymal fluid would contain whole, motile sperm with good fluid volume. Though most don't consider the impact of fluid volume, a preliminary review of our own data suggests that having moderate to copious fluid flowing out of the open epididymal tubule is a favorable finding. It makes sense that a good flow of epididymal fluid will more likely keep the intussuscepted tubule open as compared to those where sperm are seen, but there is almost no to minimal epididymal

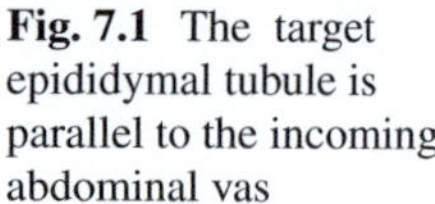

Fig. 7.1 The target epididymal tubule is parallel to the incoming abdominal vas

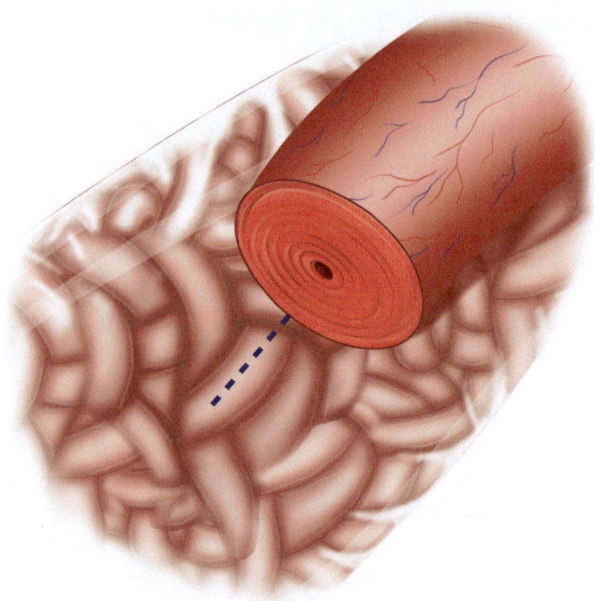

fluid. The ideal epididymal tubule for a vasoepididymostomy contains murky to white, watery, moderate to copious fluid volume with whole, motile sperm seen in a large-diameter tubule that is located in the mid body to proximal tail of the epididymis, with a parallel orientation in line with the incoming abdominal vas (Fig. 7.1).

We have identified six factors that describe the ideal epididymal tubule for a successful VE. Three factors are descriptive of the physical characteristics of the epididymal tubule itself – the location, diameter, and orientation of the target tubule. Two factors are descriptive of the fluid within the epididymal tubules – the gross and microscopic fluid findings. The last factor is the available length and most distal location of the abdominal vas.

Physical tubule characteristics can impact on the ease or difficulty of the intussusception up into the abdominal vas.

1. The diameter of the tubule can be important, as the larger caliber tubules are technically easier to work with and intussuscept up into the lumen of the abdominal vas. The finer, more delicate tubules, which are usually higher up in the epididymis, tend to be more fragile and challenging to use for a vasoepididymostomy (Fig. 7.2).
2. The location of the tubule plays a role and should ideally be situated just above the epididymal blowout. Most often we find the blockage in the distal body or tail of the epididymis, but there are occasions when we will find no sperm in the mid-body tubules or discover that the obstruction was higher up in the body or even up in the head of the epididymis. The best results should be seen when the tubule is located as far down the epididymis as possible to allow for as much sperm maturation as possible without putting the delicate repair on undue tension.

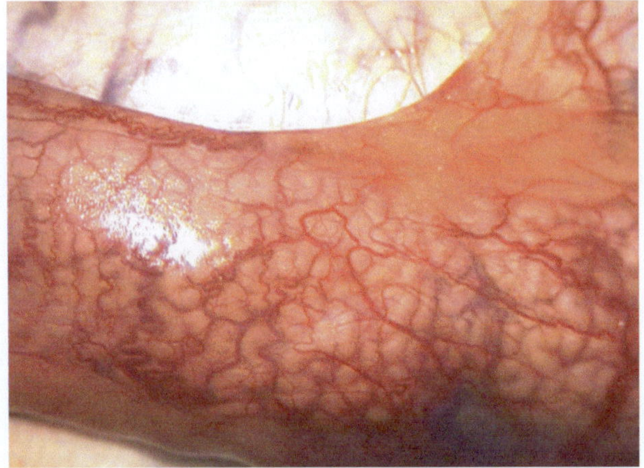

Fig. 7.2 Epididymal tubules in the body and tail tend to have a larger diameter, and so it is easier to place microsutures and intussuscept into the abdominal vasal lumen. (Photo Credit: Sheldon Marks)

Fig. 7.3 Avoid a tubule that is perpendicular to the line of the abdominal vas

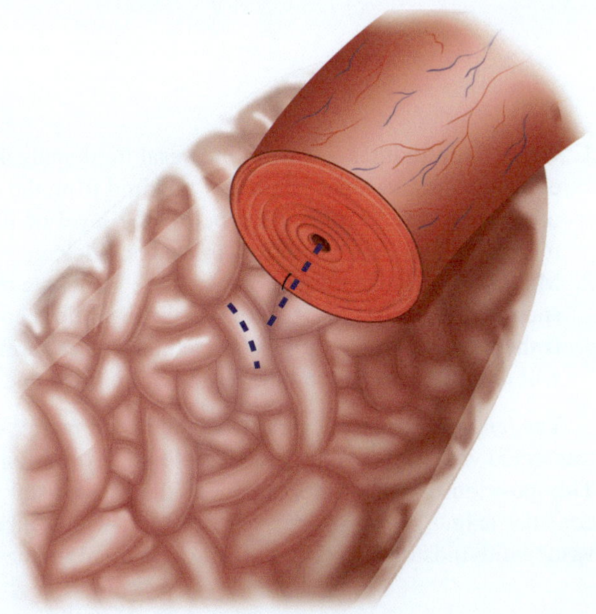

3. The orientation of the target tubule is critical for the technical tubule-to-lumen intussusception. The ideal tubule should be straight and aligned parallel and in line with the incoming secured abdominal vas to allow the open tubule to be drawn easily up and into the vasal lumen. Be careful to not use an epididymal tubule that is perpendicular to the abdominal vas (Fig. 7.3).

The *gross and microscopic tubule fluid findings* will dictate whether or not that particular tubule is acceptable for the vasoepididymostomy.

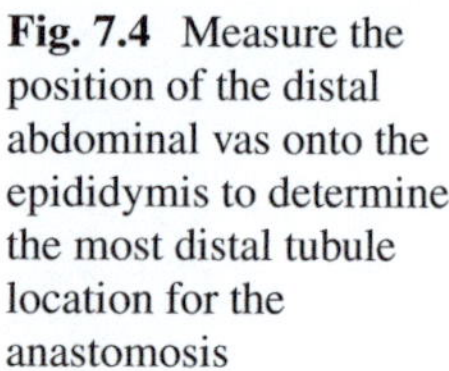

Fig. 7.4 Measure the position of the distal abdominal vas onto the epididymis to determine the most distal tubule location for the anastomosis

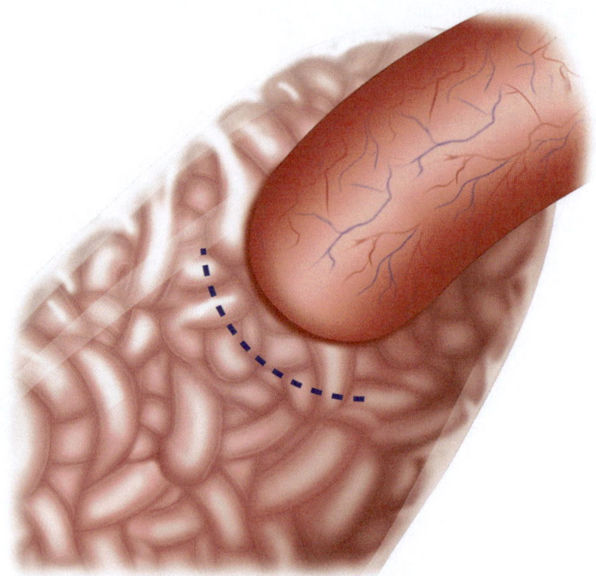

1. Gross fluid findings – as with the vasal fluid analysis, look at and document the color, consistency, and volume of the fluid from the open epididymal tubule. We often see white, creamy fluid below the level of the obstruction with clear to murky fluid within the tubules above the blockage.
2. Microscopic tubule fluid findings – look for whole motile or nonmotile sperm or sperm with partial tails. Of course, the ideal fluid contains whole, motile sperm. If there are no sperm or degenerated heads or sperm with short nubbin tails, we will move up to a new tubule to find more favorable fluid findings.

The *length of the abdominal vas* is the sixth factor, which determines where the transected vas is able to easily reach without any tension on the epididymis or repair. This position dictates the location of the most distal epididymal tubule you can consider (Fig. 7.4). A shorter vas can limit which tubule may be suitable for the vasoepididymostomy to only the more proximal tubules.

When the Open Tubule Is Not Acceptable

There are two reasons to abandon the epididymal tubule that you have just teased out and opened and move to a more cephalad tubule.(1) The epididymal fluid effluxing from the tubule defect is found on microscopic evaluation to have no sperm or sperm parts suggesting a lack of continuity with higher tubules with sperm, or (2) the defect in the epididymal tubule is significantly off-center in the lateral aspect of the tubule, is irregular, or is lengthy which would make the defect opening extend partially outside of the intussusception (Fig. 7.5).

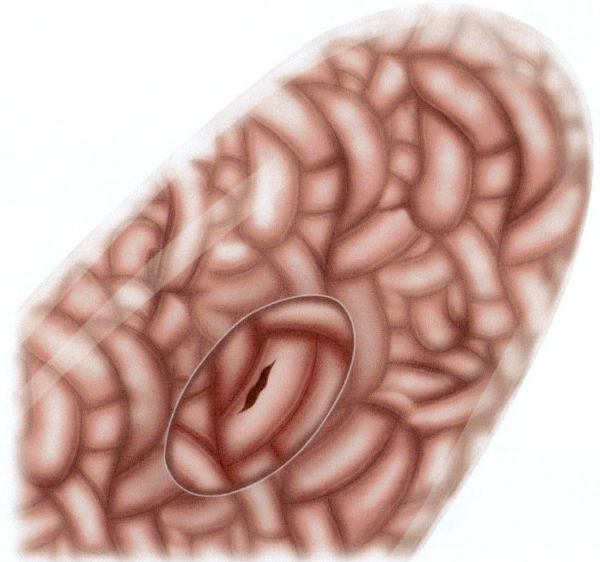

Fig. 7.5 Avoid the use of an off-center, irregular, or lengthy defect in the epididymal tubule

When you discover that the first epididymal tubule is not acceptable, most commonly because there are no sperm seen in the fluid, which suggests that the tubule is below the obstruction, then you will need to reassess the epididymis and identify a new tubule that meets the criteria, usually a few mm more proximally. If that tubule also does not have sperm or sperm parts, or there are technical issues, then you should look for another tubule, and repeat the process of teasing out and opening the tubule until you identify a tubule with acceptable fluid. This can be tedious and time-consuming. The other reason to abandon a tubule is that the defect is not acceptable. The most common reason is that the tubule tears during the teasing off of overlying adherent tissue or from overly aggressive incision or excision of the epididymal defect.

To select subsequent tubules, we often look for a difference in the gross fluid appearance within the tubule from the initial unsatisfactory tubule to suggest that the new tubule has more favorable fluid. Of course, there is no way to know until you take the time to tease out, open the tubule, and microscopically analyze the tubule fluid. Many times it may take several attempts to find a tubule that is acceptable. The concern is that the higher you move up, the less epididymis will be available to allow for sperm maturation before passing into the vas. A VE at a very high tubule near the head of the epididymis may be the reason when we achieve good sperm counts post vasoepididymostomy but with very low or no sperm motility.

Preparation of the Abdominal Vas

Transect the abdominal vas with angled Marks Vas Cutting Forceps (ASSI) so that the most superior distal portion of the vas extends out over the open epididymal tubule, allowing the vas to "lay down" over the defect and providing a larger

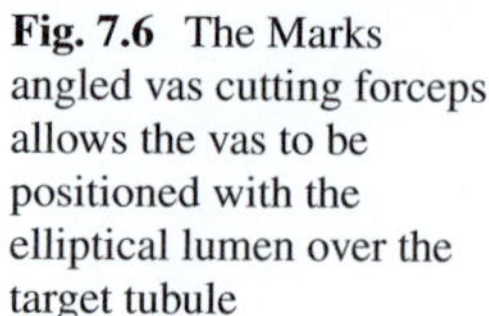

Fig. 7.6 The Marks angled vas cutting forceps allows the vas to be positioned with the elliptical lumen over the target tubule

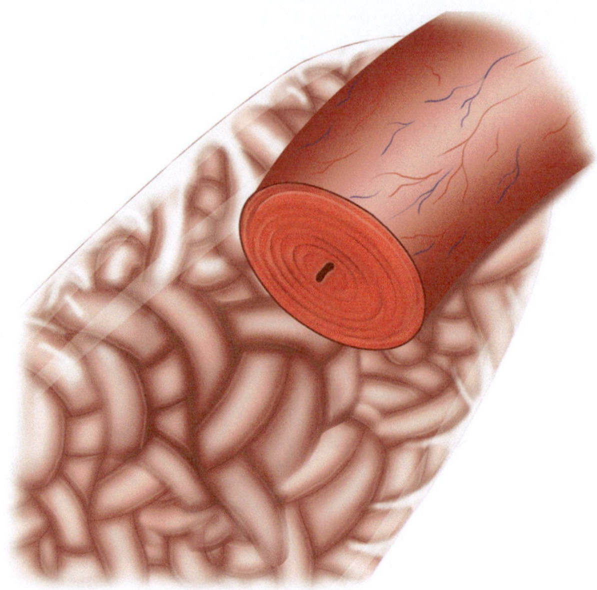

elliptical lumen for the intussusception (Fig. 7.6). As described with the vasovasostomy, next confirm patency of the abdominal vas.

Confirm Distal Vas Position over the Epididymis

Mobilize the abdominal vas and gently pull it cephalad to see where it "naturally" can reach along the epididymis without undue tension. Then position the testicle so that you can see where the end of the vas aligns with the epididymis. This allows you to identify a region of tubules above which the repair can be performed and below which there would be concerns over undue tension or a high-riding testicle. I usually mark the lowest location where the vas can reach with a line or row of dots on the epididymis with the blunt marking pen, so I don't inadvertently select a tubule too far down when working under the microscope.

Delivery of Target Tubule

Under the surgical microscope at high power, look at the underlying tubules through the usually clear to opaque epididymal tunic. Most often you will be able to see any change in diameter of the tubules and the color of the fluid within. This can be very challenging if there is thick or dense scar overlying the epididymis. It can also be just as difficult if there is significant vascularity in the epididymal tunica. The trick is to find the best tubule, correctly oriented in a window without overlying blood vessels.

Score the Epididymal Tunica and Tease Out the Tubule

Use the tip of one arm of the finest microscissors to very gently score the outer tunica (Fig. 7.7) so that the tunical window is incised in line with the tubule and the incoming abdominal vas. Then, under the highest power of the surgical microscope, very gently open the tunica along the scored line, and bluntly spread the tissues with the tips of the microscissors to free up and expose the underlying target tubule. When done correctly, the tubule will then usually protrude from the other adjacent tubules (Fig. 7.8). It may help to gently pinch the epididymis just below the window between the thumb and forefinger to help the tubule to protrude.

Beware Tearing the Tubule

Teasing out the target tubule is often very challenging as the tubule can easily tear, especially if the tubule is very fragile or there is peritubular scarring. Sometimes the tubule may be adherent to the overlying tunica which can lead to damage to the chosen tubule. Even the simple motion of wiping or dabbing the tubule with an eye spear can be enough to tear open the tubule, leaving a ragged defect often lateral to the tubule, rendering it unusable for the anastomosis. If the tubule tears, on rare occasions, the inadvertent defect may be the correct size and location, so inspect the

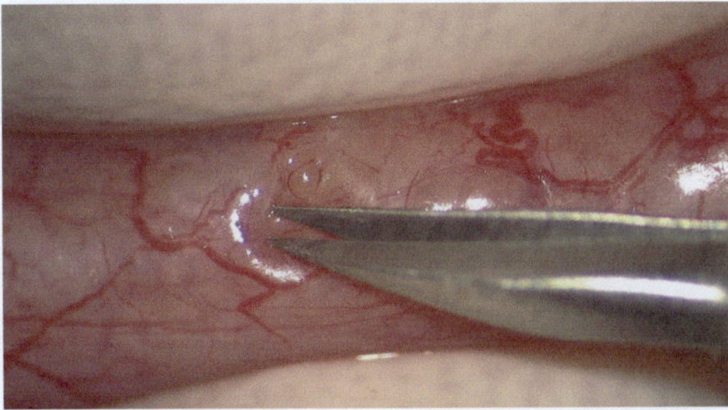

Fig. 7.7 Use the tip of one arm of the finest microscissors to very gently score the outer tunica in line with the tubule and the incoming abdominal vas. (Photo Credit: Sheldon Marks)

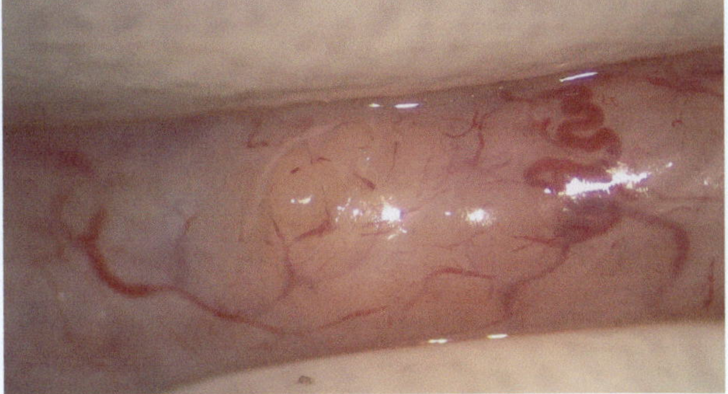

Fig. 7.8 When the target tubule is freed up, it should protrude from the other adjacent tubules. (Photo Credit: Sheldon Marks)

open to determine if you can still use it for the anastomosis. More often though, the tear renders that specific tubule unusable even if the fluid is favorable, and so you have to repeat the entire process a few mm up the epididymis, reidentifying and teasing out a new target tubule.

Tubule Position in the Tunica Window

The selected tubule should be located at the center of the tunical window (Fig. 7.9) and not off to the side near the edge of the window. A centrally located tubule makes placing the microsutures and drawing the tubule into the vasal lumen much easier. We have found that if the open tubule is located off to the side and not centrally located, the tubule can withdraw a few mm or more back under the tunica, making subsequent visualization of the tubule as well as confirming the position of location of each suture and continuing the anastomosis more difficult. If the open tubule does migrate under the tunica, regrasp the epididymis below the defect between the thumb and forefinger, and gently squeeze and relax back and forth to move the open tubule back into the center of the window.

Fig. 7.9 The selected tubule should be located at the center of the tunica window and not off to the side, near, or under the edge of the window

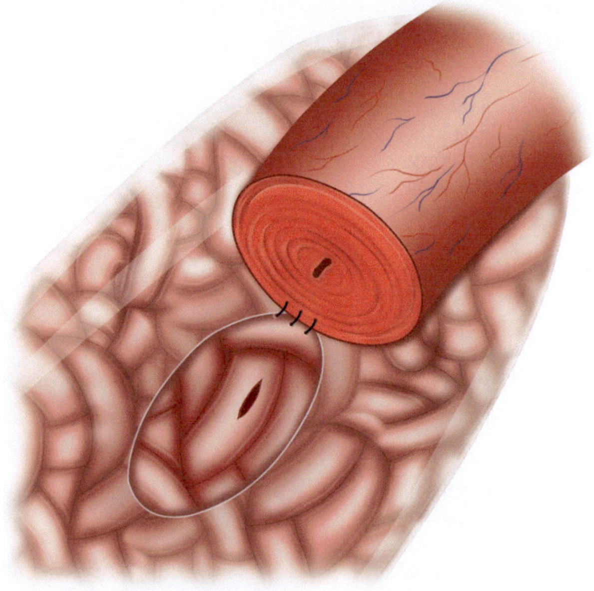

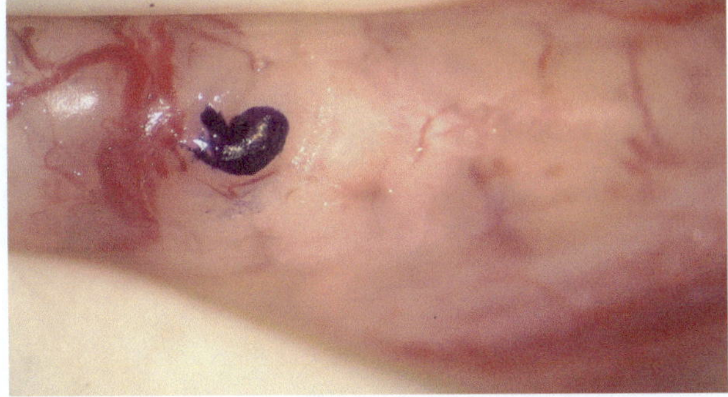

Fig. 7.10 Ink the arch of the target tubule with a blunt-tipped marking pen so that when incised the mucosal edge of the defect will be clearly defined. (Photo Credit: Sheldon Marks)

Ink the Arch of the Tubule

With the overlying tissues teased off of the clean tubule, which is now protruding out of the window, dab the top of the tubule with a dry eye spear, and ink the arch of the target tubule with a blunt-tipped marking pen (Fig. 7.10). Be extremely careful as the act of placing the ink can also disrupt and tear the tubule. The inking of the tubule dramatically improves your ability to visualize the more defined mucosal edge of the tubule defect. If there is a low volume of the epididymal fluid, then the opened tubule can collapse on itself, and the edges of the defect can become very difficult to see.

Opening the Tubule: Incise Versus Excise Ellipse

There are two primary techniques for creating the window in the epididymal tubule, with pros and cons to each. The first and most commonly used technique is to partially pass the 70 micron needles from two separate short 2.5 inch 10-0 Nylon suture through the target tubule so that the needles are parallel to each other and the tubule, extending out on both sides of the tubule with a bridge of tubule between (Fig. 7.11). The arch of the tubule between the needles is then incised longitudinally with the tip of a 5 mm 15 degree micro-ophthalmic blade (ASSI.KA155) (Fig. 7.12) to create the tubulotomy. The needles are then drawn out of the tissue so that half of the suture length is on either side of the tubule (Fig. 7.13). The advantage to this technique is that the tubule usually remains plump and distended, and so it is easier to precisely place both of the microneedles. The disadvantage is that you now have the tiny microsutures barely attached through a minimal layer of tubule that can easily

Fig. 7.11 Pass the 70 micron needles through the target tubule so that the needles are parallel to each other and the tubule, extending out on both sides of the tubule with a bridge of tubule between

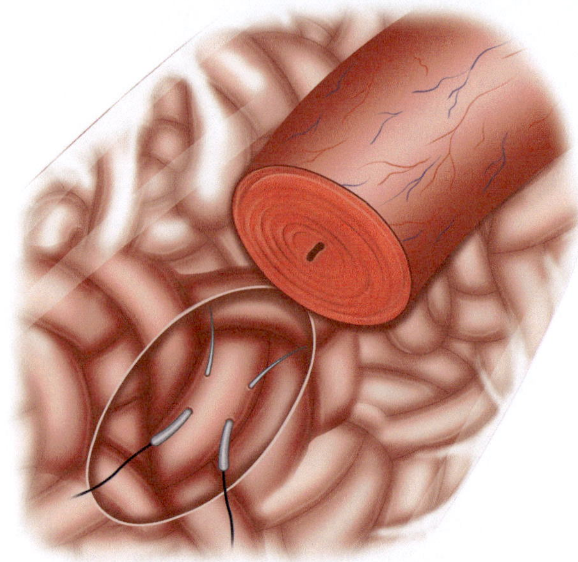

Fig. 7.12 Incise the arch of the epididymal tubule longitudinally with a micro-ophthalmic blade

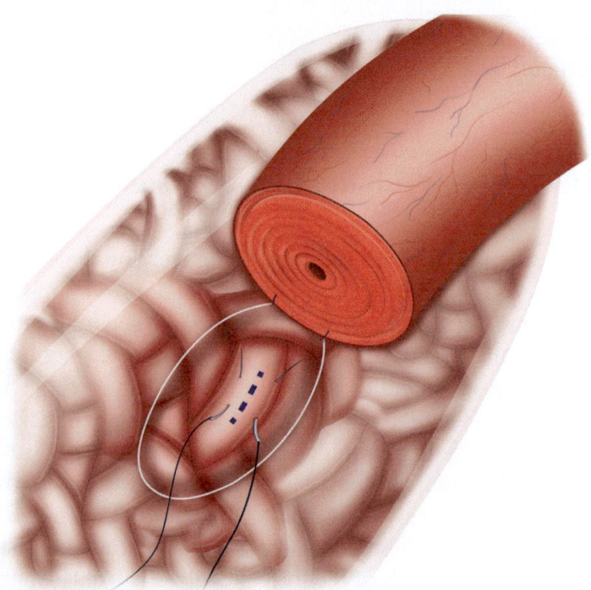

be torn if the sutures are pulled. Just as frustrating, sometimes the sutures can become tangled with each other or the needles inadvertently pulled off. Another disadvantage to this technique is that if the tubule fluid is not acceptable then both needles need to be backed out and then safely secured until they are used again for the next tubule. This can cause problems with the delicate 70 micron needles if you

Fig. 7.13 The microneedles are then drawn out of the tissue so that half of the suture length is on either side of the tubule

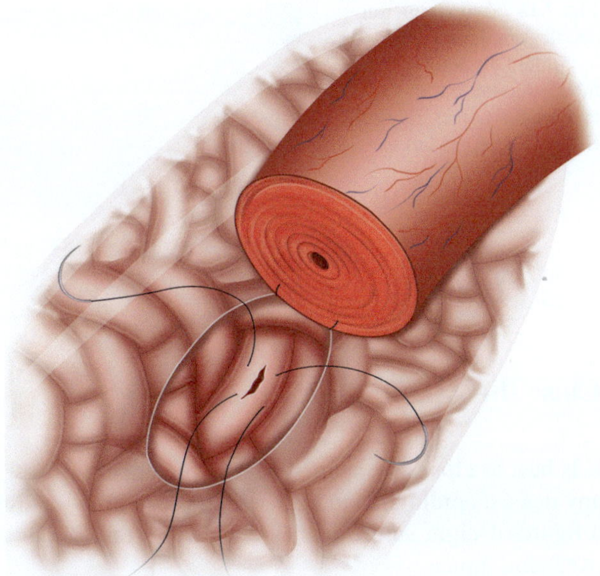

Fig. 7.14 Excision of a small longitudinal ellipse in the arch of the target tubule with very fine microscissors. (Photo Credit: Sheldon Marks)

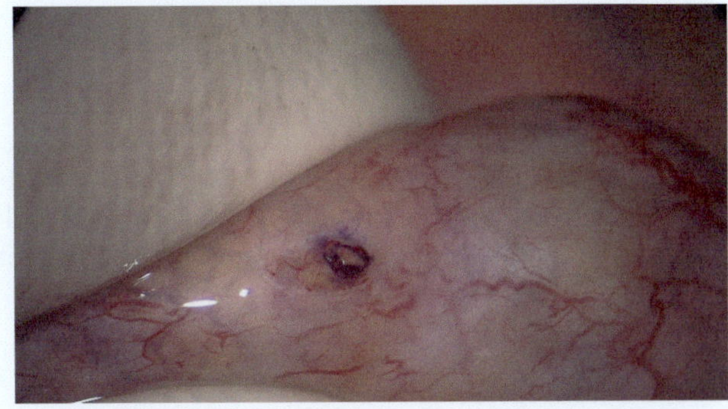

have to place and then remove them on several tubules until you find one that has favorable fluid.

The other approach, which I prefer, is to excise a small longitudinal ellipse in the arch of the target tubule with very fine microscissors, such as the Lipshultz epididymovasostomy dissecting scissors (ASSI SDC15RVL) (Fig. 7.14). The 70 micron needles from two separate 2.5 inch 10-0 nylon sutures are then placed longitudinally, through the tubule, lateral to the epididymal defect (Fig. 7.15). The advantage is that there is less handling of the delicate 70 micron needles if that tubule is found to be unsatisfactory for the repair. The downside to this technique is that the tubule is collapsed after the window is excised, and so many can find it more difficult to accurately place the 70 micron needles through the tubules lateral to the excised ellipse.

Fig. 7.15 Two 70 micron needles are then placed longitudinally though the tubule, lateral to the epididymal defect. (Photo Credit: Sheldon Marks)

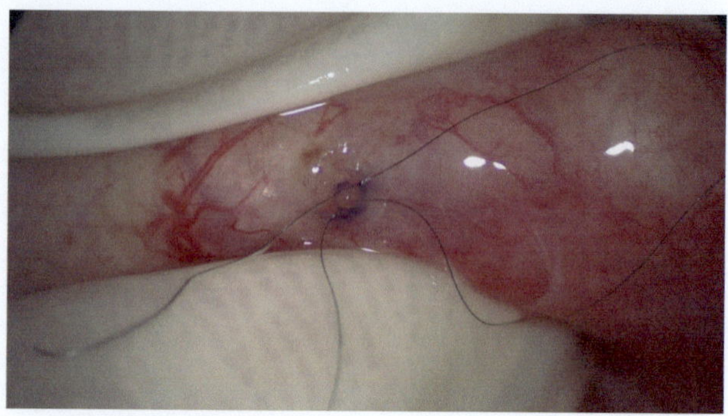

Close the Abandoned, Unusable Tubule

It is best to close any opened but unacceptable tubules. You can close the defect of any unused epididymal tubules with pulses of low-energy bipolar and/or, as I prefer, a figure-of-eight suture with 9-0 suture in the tubule and a 7-0 nylon closing the overlying tunica.

Epididymal Fluid Analysis

The gross and microscopic analysis of the fluid from the opened epididymal tubule will help you to identify a tubule that will be acceptable for the intussusception. Many times, the epididymal fluid will have whole and even motile sperm, while other instances there may be no sperm or only debris noted.

Gross Description

As with the vasal fluid, note and record the volume, color, and consistency of the fluid effluxing from the epididymal tubule and each additional tubule that you may have to open. There are times when the fluid may be of good volume initially and then become minimal. The fluid can be clear, murky, white, yellow, or brown.

Microscopic Findings

As soon as the tubule is opened, touch the end of a sterile glass slide onto the open tubule to obtain a drop of the fluid for microscopic analysis. The analysis of the slide to look for sperm or sperm parts can be done either at the adjacent microscope by the surgeon or assistant or by handing the slide to an andrologist who can analyze the fluid under a high-power lab microscope. Having the andrologist do this analysis allows the surgeon to continue with the surgery and not have to stop and take the time to look at the slide. Once adequate sperm are seen, you can proceed with the anastomosis. I consider the fluid to be acceptable if there are whole sperm or even just sperm with partial tails, which is consistent with an open system. There are some experts that will only use that tubule if they see whole sperm, and some require complete, motile sperm in the fluid, which allows for sperm banking as well. As the chances for success and pregnancy are lower with a VE, having cryopreserved sperm as backup in this situation is even more important for some surgeons and patients. If the epididymal fluid is bankable, then aspirate with HTF, and deliver to the andrologist for cryopreservation.

Setting Up the Intussusception

Senior reversal experts will tell you that the most difficult aspect of any vasoepididymostomy is usually the setup. Finding and bringing together the vas to the correct epididymal tubule is the main challenge and sometimes the most time-consuming aspect of the reversal on that side. One of the most challenging aspects to a VE is getting enough abdominal vasal length and securing the vas to be able to bring the vas down to the target epididymal tubule without any traction or drawing the testicle higher up into the scrotum, a guaranteed way to have an unhappy patient. When the abdominal vas is transected above the vasectomy scar, it is important to preserve as much abdominal length as possible. The trick is to be as close to the vasal defect as you can while not having any visible vasal damage or scarring from the vasectomy. Many times, the first challenge is prepping and positioning the abdominal vas for the VE. Once the vas is prepped and secured down to the acceptable epididymal tubule, then the microsurgery becomes routine as you go step by step to perform the vasoepididymostomy. Finding the correct epididymal tubule can be a frustrating and time-consuming part of a vasoepididymostomy. The goal is to find the ideal tubule in the best location with favorable intratubular fluid characteristics and sperm. With a VE there are often dilemmas and competing challenges.

Securing the Vas Through the Tunica Vaginalis

Push the tip of a microhemostat up through the most superior aspect of the tunica vaginalis, with care to avoid any blood vessels. Grasp the adventitia around the transected end of the abdominal vas with the microhemostat, and draw the vas through the tunnel of the tunica vaginalis (Fig. 7.16). Control any bleeding noted at the tunica window now rather than wait until later when it may be more difficult to visualize any bleeding sites. Secure the adventitia and superficial muscularis of the

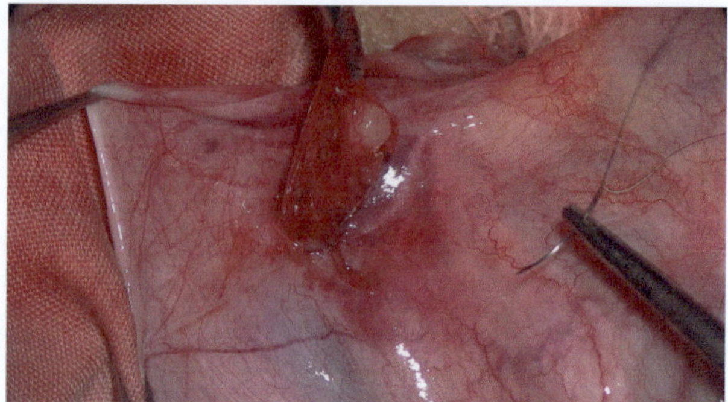

Fig. 7.16 The adventitia around the transected end of the abdominal vas is grasped with the microhemostat and the vas drawn through the tunnel of the tunica vaginalis. (Photo Credit: Sheldon Marks)

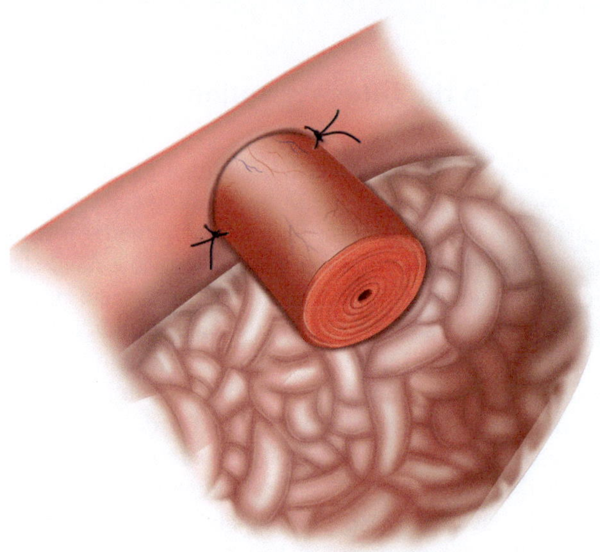

Fig. 7.17 The adventitia and superficial muscularis of the vas are secured with 7-0 nylon to the edges of the tunica vaginalis defect at 3 and 9 o'clock position

vas to the edges of the tunica vaginalis defect at 3 and 9 o'clock position with interrupted 7-0 nylon sutures (Fig. 7.17). Then secure the vas to the underlying tunica in several more locations with 7-0 nylon interrupted stitches to prevent any traction on the repair and to position the transected face of the abdominal vas up to the open tubule. Ideally the face of the abdominal vas should be positioned so that it lies just at and over the open epididymal tubule (Fig. 7.18).

You can bring the abdominal vas down through the tunica earlier, but if you are doing this before you expose and open the tubule, it is best not to secure the vas past the defect in the superior tunica until you have confirmed that the epididymal fluid is favorable with sperm from the specific tubule that you plan to use. Then you can place the securing sutures to align the abdominal vas up to the open tubule. Though you can secure the vas through and along the tunica earlier, the concern is that if you need to move up several cm along the epididymis to higher tubules, you may have to cut the reinforcing sutures and resecure the abdominal vas to the higher tubule location.

Fig. 7.18 The face of the
abdominal vas should be
positioned so that it lies
just at the open epididymal
tubule

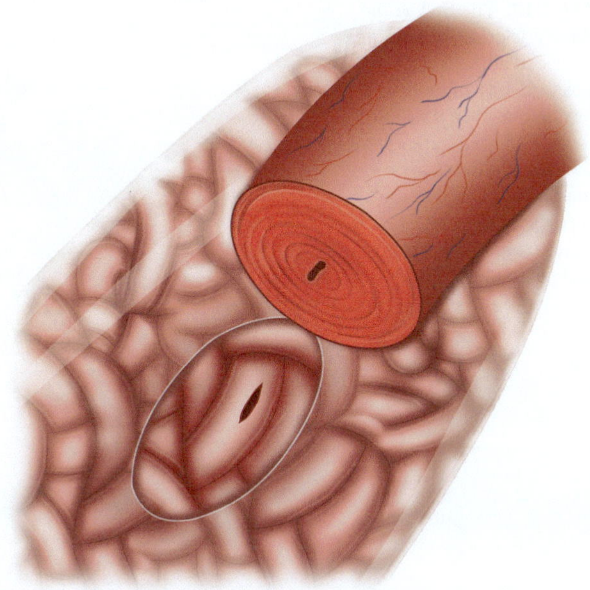

Securing the Posterior Vas to the Epididymal Tunica

Once the abdominal vas is secured in position over the open tubule, then place the first of three interrupted 9-0 nylon sutures, approximating the superficial muscularis of the posterior abdominal vas to the corresponding inferior position of the edge of the window in the epididymal tunica below the open tubule. The first of the three posterior wall sutures is placed at the 6 o'clock position passing the needle out-to-in through the tunica and then in the vasal lumen and out the superficial muscularis and then tied (Fig. 7.19). Then place and tie the two additional sutures in a similar fashion at the 4 and 8 o'clock positions. This should then have the face of the vas secured up to and positioned almost over the epididymal tubule.

Timing of the Epididymal Tubule Suture Placement

As was noted, if you placed the short double- armed 10-0 sutures early when you created the defect in the tubule, then there is the possibility that the sutures can be inadvertently pulled and break, pop the needle off, or tear the tubule, forcing you to start the process over again sometimes with a new tubule. In addition, the microsutures can become tangled with normal irrigation or manipulation and preparation of the vas to the epididymis. If you postpone placing the epididymal sutures until after the posterior wall 9-0 sutures securing the abdominal vas are placed and tied, then often you may have pulled down the tunica of the epididymis, changing the angle of

Fig. 7.19 The first of the three posterior wall sutures is placed at the 6 o'clock position, passing the needle out-to-in through the epididymal tunica into the defect created over the tubule and then into the superficial muscularis at the corresponding position and out

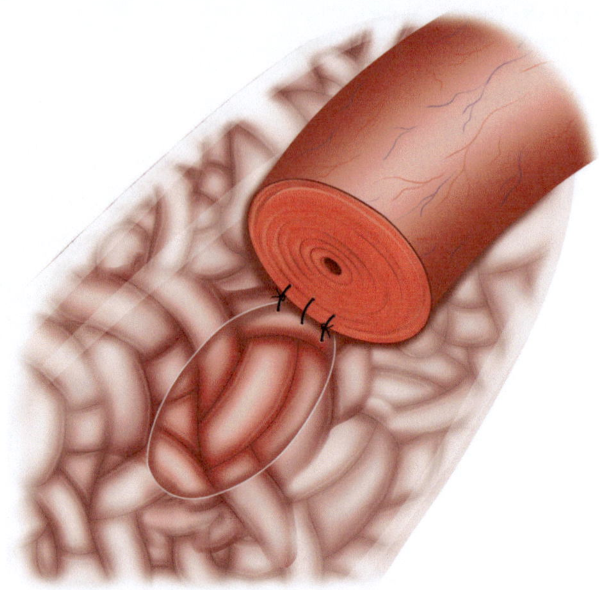

the tubule, which can make visualization of the epididymal defect and the placement and tying of the microsutures and subsequent intussusception more challenging.

VE Suture and Needle Selection

If the sutures are not already placed as part of the tubule incision, then for the longitudinal intussusception technique, we have found that the ideal sutures are the 2.5 cm 10-0 nylon double-armed sutures with 70 micron bicurve needles with M.E.T.$_{TM}$ points (Sharpoint $_{TM}$ AA-2492). Over the years we have not been satisfied with trials with a number of other needle and suture options. The unique design of the bicurve angle of the 70 micron needle is found to pass easily into the vasal lumen and out through the vasal mucosa and muscularis as well as the epididymal tubule.

Passage of 10-0 Sutures Through the Vasal Mucosa

Once you have confirmed that the abdominal vas is correctly positioned and secured on no traction, pass the needle on the 10-0 sutures into the vasal lumen. Pass the needle of the 10–0 up and into the vasal lumen mucosa 1–2 mm in from the edge and then out through the vasal muscularis. The needles should all exit at the junction of the inner one-third and outer two-thirds of the muscularis. Preplaced microdots can help with the accurate placement of the needles (Fig. 7.20).

I prefer to start with the two posterior epididymal sutures at the 4 o'clock and then the 8 o'clock position and then place the anterior sutures at 10 o'clock and then the 2 o'clock position. These sutures will draw the open loop of tubule up and into the lumen to open and separate the edges. Others will place the 8 o'clock and 10 o'clock sutures first and then the opposite side 4 o'clock and 2 o'clock sutures last (Figs. 7.21, 7.22, 7.23 and 7.24).

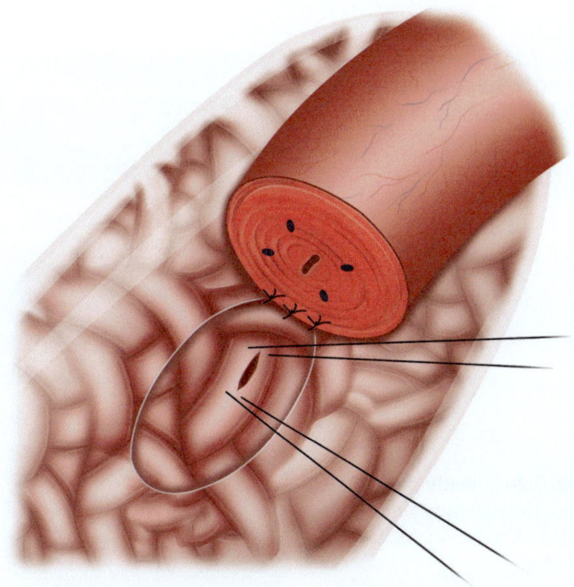

Fig. 7.20 Preplaced microdots on the abdomen vas can help with the accurate placement of the needles

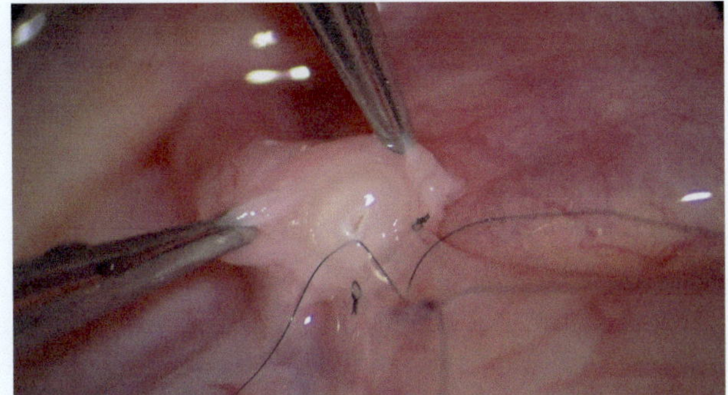

Fig. 7.21 Pass the posterior 8 o'clock epididymal needle into the corresponding location in the vasal lumen and out the muscularis. (Photo Credit: Sheldon Marks)

Fig. 7.22 Then place the 4 o'clock epididymal needle into the lumen and out. (Photo Credit: Sheldon Marks)

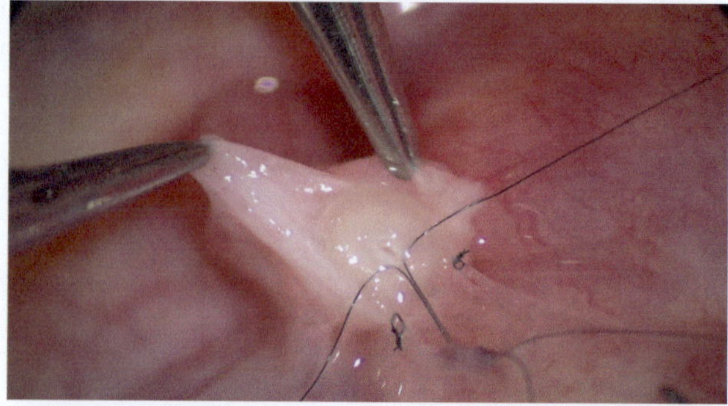

Fig. 7.23 Then pass the anterior suture at the 10 o'clock position. (Photo Credit: Sheldon Marks)

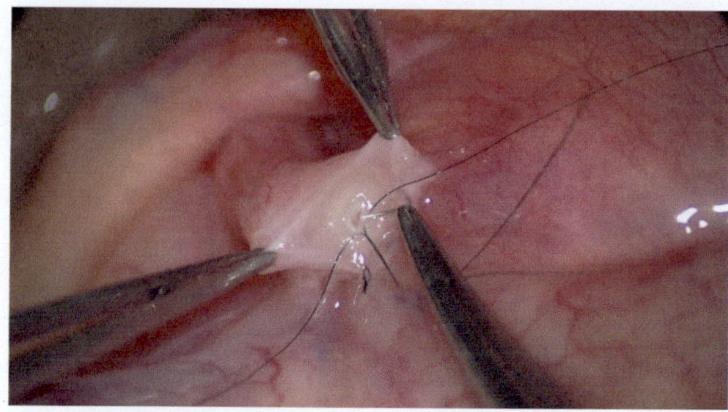

Fig. 7.24 Finally place the 2 o'clock position suture. (Photo Credit: Sheldon Marks)

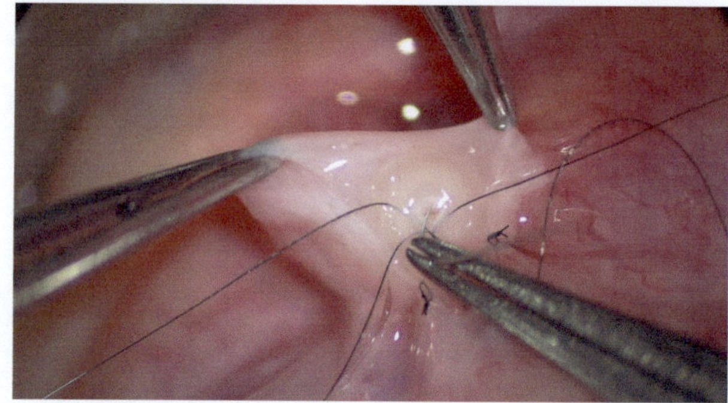

Test the Invagination of Tubule

Once all sutures are in place, to test the position and planned intussusception, then gently grasp and pull the sutures away from the vas with equal traction on both sides to be sure that the open epididymal tubule is easily drawn up and into the correct position within the open vasal lumen (Fig. 7.25). You must be extremely delicate and careful as if you grasp or pull too hard you can tear the sutures out of the epididymal tubule or break the sutures.

Fig. 7.25 Confirm that the open epididymal tubule is easily intussuscepted up and into the correct position within the open vasal lumen. (Photo Credit: Sheldon Marks)

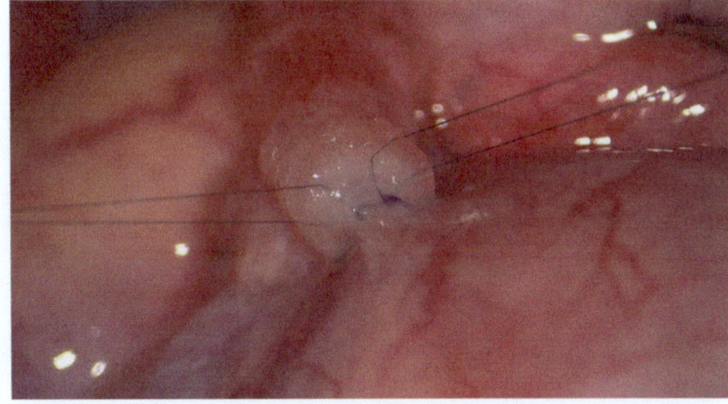

Fig. 7.26 With the open tubule up in the vasal lumen, very gently pull and tie the 2 and 4 o'clock sutures and then the 8 and 10 o'clock sutures, securing the intussuscepted tubule within the vasal lumen. (Photo Credit: Sheldon Marks)

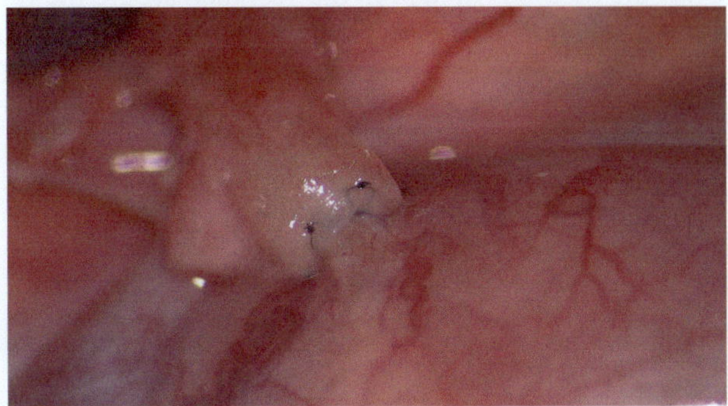

Draw and Tie the Intussusception Sutures

Carefully lift away the sutures on the proximal side to draw the open tubule into position within the open vasal lumen and then tie them down, watching to be sure the open tubule remains in position within the vasal lumen. Then repeat on the contralateral side. If there are any concerns over tension from the distal vas, then the vasal adventitia can be gently drawn up to pull the vasal lumen over the tubule as the sutures are tied (Fig. 7.26).

When a Suture Breaks

If a suture breaks on one side, either before, during, or after tying the contralateral suture, then you may be able to repass another 2.5 cm 10-0 double-armed needle longitudinally again along the side of the open epididymal tubule and then up and out the lumen. If you are unable to do this, then the alternative is to place two or three 10-0 interrupted sutures starting at edge of the epididymal tubule, out-to-in and then in-to-out through corresponding positions within the open vasal lumen to the muscularis.

If the Tubule Tears

If while gently retracting the sutures and drawing the tubule up into the open vasal lumen the tubule tears, then you have to take down any suture already placed and examine the damaged tubule to see if it is salvageable or if you have to start the entire process over with a new epididymal tubule.

Reinforce the Remaining Muscularis to the Tunica

Once the tubule is up and in the vas, then secure the remaining anterior and lateral vasal muscularis to the edges of the corresponding epididymal tunica window with interrupted 9-0 nylon sutures, again from the edge of the epididymal window to the outer third of the muscularis of the abdominal vas (Fig. 7.27).

Secure the Adventitial Layer

Reinforce the anastomosis, when possible, with additional interrupted 7-0 nylon bringing together the vasal adventitia to the adjacent epididymal tunica (Fig. 7.28). When placing these outermost sutures, it is important not to cause undue traction or twisting of the repair.

Banking of Sperm

If the patient requested banking of sperm and the fluid from the epididymal tubule was not bankable, then this is when you can perform a mini-TESE through a pinhole defect in the tunica albuginea to retrieve seminiferous tubules for cryopreservation.

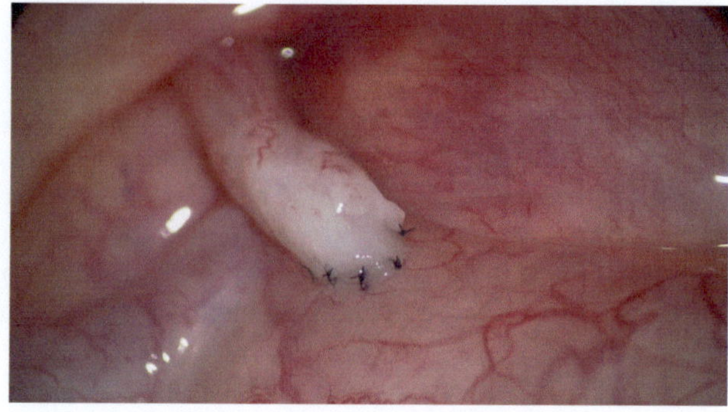

Fig. 7.27 Secure the remaining anterior and lateral vasal muscularis to the edges of the corresponding epididymal tunica window with interrupted 9-0 nylon sutures. (Photo Credit: Sheldon Marks)

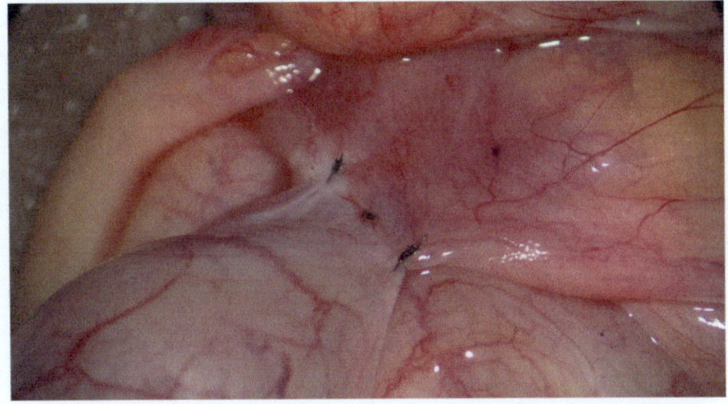

Fig. 7.28 Reinforce the anastomosis with additional interrupted 7-0 nylon, bringing together the vasal adventitia to the adjacent epididymal tunica. (Photo Credit: Sheldon Marks)

If this is the first side, then you can postpone this until you can determine if the contralateral side has bankable vasal fluid or epididymal fluid.

Close the Tunica

Before you start to close the tunica, this is the time to re-examine the defect in the tunica vaginalis for any bleeding points that need to be addressed. Re-examine the length of the vas and confirm that there is no bleeding from the anastomosis. If any bleeding sites are identified, address with pinpoint microbipolar. Then reinfiltrate the edges of the open tunica vaginalis with the lidocaine/bupivacaine anesthetic, and approximate the edges of the tunica with a running 4-0 Vicryl suture. Care should be taken not to inadvertently damage any underlying epididymal tubules and catch the underlying tunica albuginea, the epididymis, or the appendix testis in the running Vicryl suture.

Replace the Testicle

Gently return the testicle back into position in the hemiscrotum. It is important to not lift up the testicle and put the new intussusception on excessive traction and so risk damaging the repair. To do this we use small retractors to lift the skin and subcutaneous tissues at three equidistant points and then gently replace the testicle back into the hemiscrotum in correct position, superior end first.

The Five- or Six-Suture End-to-Side Vasoepididymostomy

This was the standard vasoepididymostomy technique used before the intussusception method was developed and became the primary technique for most reversal experts. There are still some experts that prefer and use this as their VE technique.

Even if you routinely use the two-suture intussusception technique, there may be situations when this technique will be useful. One reason to use the five- to six-suture anastomosis would be if the incision in the target epididymal tubule is too long and so when intussuscepted, the opening of the epididymal tubule would extend partially outside of the vasal lumen, leading to a leakage of the epididymal fluid and sperm. In this case, you have the option to start over with a new tubule, or you may want to use this technique to pass five or six separate epididymal tubule out-to-in and then in-to-out the abdominal vasal mucosa, similar to a vasovasostomy.

Set Up as with the Intussusception VE

Position and secure the vas with the setup as with the intussusception vasoepididymostomy. Draw the vas through a tunnel at the superior aspect of the tunica vaginalis, and secure the abdominal vas through and along the tunica with interrupted 7-0 nylon sutures. Then identify, tease out, and open the epididymal tubule. Once you have confirmed that the fluid and tubule are favorable, then secure the vas in multiple positions so that the abdominal vas is just up to and just over the open epididymal tubule. Then place the three interrupted posterior 9-0 sutures to secure the inferior aspect of the epididymal tunica window to the posterior muscularis of the abdominal vas to secure and position the vas over the open tubule.

Place Five or Six of the 10-0 Sutures

Place five or six of the 10-0 epididymal sutures, with the number dictated by the size of the defect in the epididymal tubule. What differs is that with this technique you would place the first mucosal out-to-in 10-0 nylon suture with the bicurve 70 micron needle through the 6 o'clock position of the tubulotomy. Repeat the placement of the next two mucosal sutures at the 4 and 8 o'clock positions (Fig. 7.29). You can use separate double-armed short sutures or a long 10-0 on a 70 micron needle with each suture placed and then cut and tied.

Place Mucosal Sutures into the Vasal Mucosa

Next pass the needles of these three sutures into the vasal mucosa lumen at corresponding positions and out the muscularis, just as with the intussusception technique. Once they are placed, then tie all three, starting with the 6 o'clock suture, and then tie the two lateral sutures to draw the inferior aspect of the open tubule up to the abdominal lumen mucosa.

Test the Repair and Tie the Sutures

Then place but not tie the 2, 10, and 12 o'clock sutures through the epididymal tubule and then out the vasal lumen mucosa until all are placed. Once you have placed the sutures on gentle traction and confirmed that they do easily draw down to the vasal mucosa, then tie the lateral sutures, and then finish with the 12 o'clock suture (Fig. 7.30). For a smaller tubular defect, you can use a total of five equidistant 10-0 sutures.

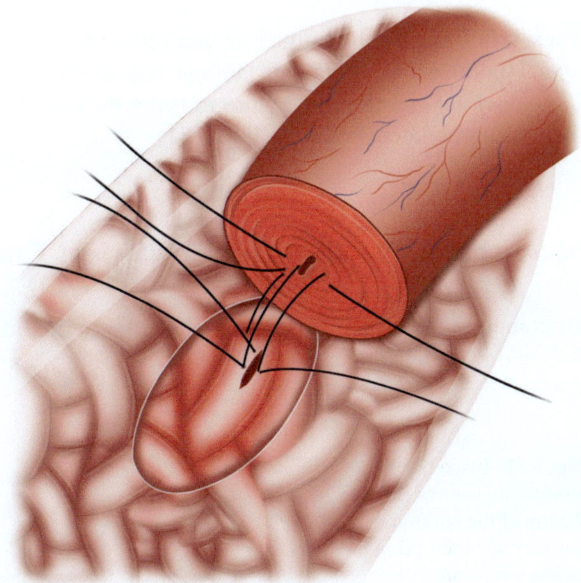

Fig. 7.29 For the standard five- to six-suture end-to-side VE, after the posterior 9-0 sutures are placed, pass the mucosal out-to-in 10-0 suture with the bicurve 70 micron needle through the 6, 4, and 8 o'clock position of the tubulotomy

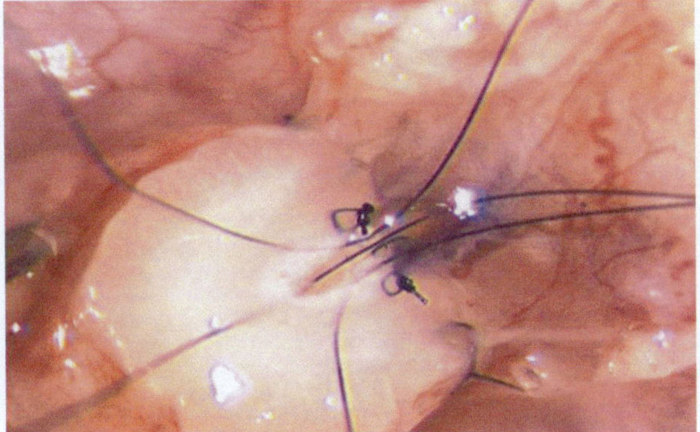

Fig. 7.30 Place and then tie the 2, 10, and 12 o'clock 10-0 nylon sutures through the epididymal tubule and then out the vasal lumen mucosa

If a Suture Breaks or the Mucosa Tears

When possible try to replace the suture in the gap left by the broken suture. This can be difficult if it is the last suture to tie so there is minimal visible gap and it can be difficult to precisely place the needle. If the mucosa of the tubule tears, then you will have to replace the suture adjacent to the tear.

Reinforce the Muscularis to the Tunica

Then reinforce the remainder of the circumference with interrupted epididymal tunica to muscularis 9-0 nylon sutures, tied as each is placed. One tip is to place the 12 o'clock 9-0 reinforcing suture to bring the top of the anastomosis together and then fill in the lateral sutures (Fig. 7.31).

Secure the Adventitia to the Epididymal Tunica

To complete the repair, secure the adventitia to epididymal tunica with interrupted 7-0 nylon when technically possible to reduce any tension on the anastomosis.

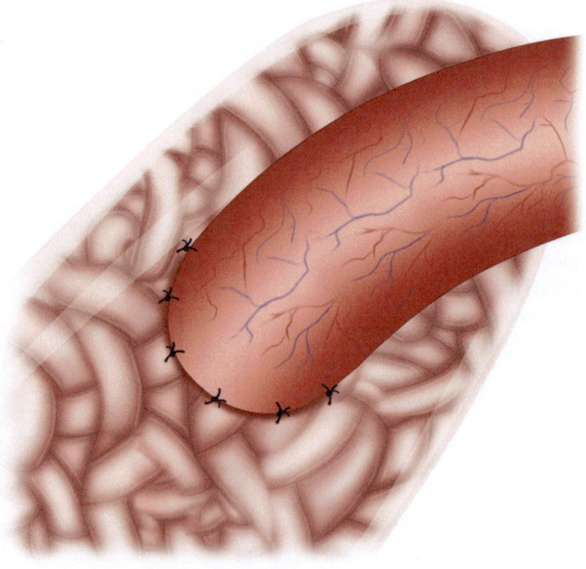

Fig. 7.31 Place the 9-0 reinforcing sutures to bring the top of the anastomosis together and then fill in the lateral 9-0 sutures

Close the Tunica and Replace the Testicle

Confirm that there is no bleeding and that the vasoepididymostomy is intact, infiltrate with local anesthesia, and close the tunica and gently replace the testicle back into the hemiscrotum, being careful not to place the anastomosis on undue traction. As with the intussusception technique, direct the superior aspect of the testicle into the defect to minimize any tension.

References

1. Chawla A, O'Brien J, Lisi M, et al. Should all urologists performing vasectomy reversals be able to perform vasoepididymostomies if required? J Urol. 2004;172:1048–50.
2. Crain DS, Roberts JL, Amling CL. Practice patterns in vasectomy reversal surgery: results of a questionnaire study among practicing urologists. J Urol. 2004;171:311–5.
3. Chan PT. The evolution and refinement of vasoepididymostomy techniques. Asian J Androl. 2013;15:49–55. Asian J Androl 2016 Jan-Feb; 18(1): 129–133.
4. Ostrowski KA, Tadros NN, Polackwich AS, McClure RD, Fuchs EF, Hedges JC. Factors and practice patterns that affect the decision for vasoepididymostomy. Can J Urol. 2017;24(1):8651–5.
5. Fuchs ME, Anderson RE, Ostrowski KA, Brant WO, Fuchs EF. Pre-operative risk factors associated with need for vasoepididymostomy at the time of vasectomy reversal. Andrology. 2016;4(1):160–2.
6. Matthews GJ, Schlegel PN, Goldstein M. Patency following microsurgical vasoepididymostomy and vasovasostomy: temporal considerations. J Urol. 1995;154:2070–3.
7. Kumar R, Gautam G, Gupta NP. Early patency rates after the two-suture invagination technique of vaso-epididymal anastomosis for idiopathic obstruction. BJU Int. 2006;97:575–7.
8. Peng J, Yuan Y, Zhang Z, Gao B, Song W, et al. Patency rates of microsurgical vasoepididymostomy for patients with idiopathic obstructive azoospermia: a prospective analysis of factors associated with patency – single-center experience. Urology. 2012;79:119–22.
9. Chan PT, Brandell RA, Goldstein M. Prospective analysis of outcomes after microsurgical intussusception vasoepididymostomy. BJU Int. 2005;96:598–601.

Chapter 8
Intraoperative Dilemmas and Challenges with Vasovasostomy and Vasoepididymostomy

There are many anatomic and surgical challenges that the urologic microsurgeon will encounter when performing vasectomy reversals. This section discusses a few of the unique and challenging dilemmas that you may unexpectedly encounter during a vasectomy reversal, whether vasovasostomy or vasoepididymostomy. These include having to modify techniques to address a protuberant, pouchy abdominal vasal mucosa, performing the anastomosis down to the thin-walled, deep convoluted testicular vas, an absent peri-vasal adventitia, or a large epididymal cyst. More commonly you will encounter widely discrepant vasal lumens which can be challenging to perform a watertight anastomosis even for the most experienced microsurgeons. Vasoepididymostomy specific challenges include the absence of fluid or sperm in the open epididymal tubules; a very vascular or heavily scarred overlying epididymal tunica obscuring the underlying tubules; the presence of only flat, almost nonvisible epididymal tubules; as well as having to perform the repair on no tension with a lengthy vasal gap.

Pouchy Abdominal Mucosa

The finding of a pouchy mucosa seen protruding out of the abdominal lumen is unacceptable for the anastomosis, and so the vas must be recut a few mm up the vas (Fig. 8.1). This protuberant mucosa makes it very difficult to clearly visualize the edges and so accurately place the mucosal sutures. Not only is this a challenge to perform, but there are significantly increased risks for accidentally catching the opposing wall with the needle and inadvertently sewing the lumen shut. When you retransect the vas, be sure the vas is not on any superior or lateral traction. Sometimes it may take several recuts to find the vas with normal mucosa that does not protrude.

© Springer Nature Switzerland AG 2019
S. H. F. Marks, *Vasectomy Reversal*,
https://doi.org/10.1007/978-3-030-00455-2_8

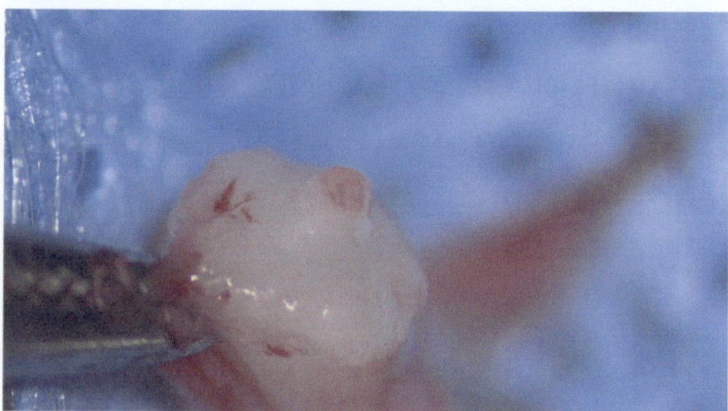

Fig. 8.1 Pouchy, protuberant mucosa from abdominal vasal lumen. (Photo Credit: Sheldon Marks)

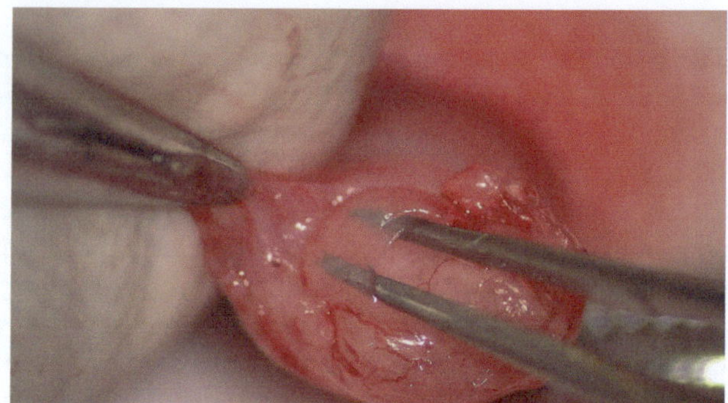

Fig. 8.2 The thin and sometimes almost minimal muscularis layer of the testicular deep convoluted vas

Deep Convoluted Vas

When the transected end of the testicular vas is located down in the deep convoluted portion, this can create additional challenges to the repair. We have previously addressed the importance of identifying a central lumen, which is often difficult to do in the deep convoluted vas. From a technical point of view, the anastomosis is significantly more challenging, as you have to approximate together the thick multiple muscularis layers of the abdominal vas to a very thin and sometimes almost minimal muscularis layer of the testicular deep convoluted vas (Fig. 8.2). There are times when performing this repair can seem more like an intussusception VE, as you try to anastomose the tip of a very fine convoluted vas up to the much larger-diameter abdominal vasal lumen. For the most extreme cases, the easiest portion starts with the lumen-to-lumen sutures, and then the challenge is to reinforce the muscularis layers as best you can (Fig. 8.3) [1, 2].

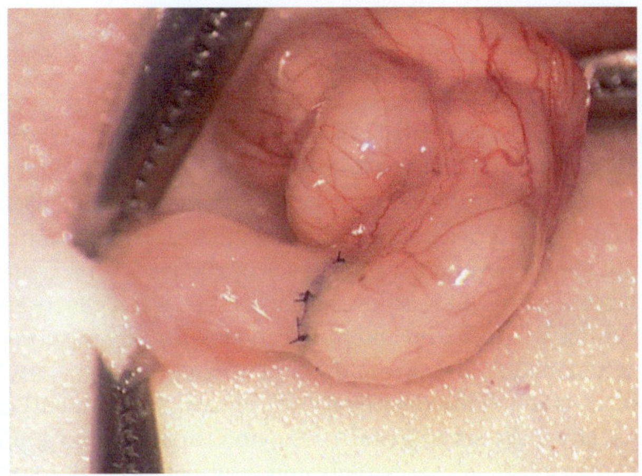

Fig. 8.3 Reinforcing the muscularis layers with a deep convoluted vasovasostomy. (Photo Credit: Sheldon Marks)

Absent Peri-vasal Adventitia

There are times when there is no usable peri-vasal adventitia for the outermost layer in a multilayer VV. If you feel additional sutures are needed to reduce any tension on the repair, when possible you can place interrupted 7-0 nylon sutures through just the edge of the muscularis in the abdominal and testicular vas. Sometimes you do not have enough adventitial tissue and so will have to settle for a two-layer closure.

Epididymal Cyst/Spermatocele

The presence of an epididymal cyst can impact on the outcomes of the vasovasostomy or vasoepididymostomy and decision-making as it may function as a decompressing path of least resistance for the sperm. Epididymal cysts can be single or multiple and very small up to very large. For large cysts that are painful to the patient, we have not had great results with simple aspiration of the cyst fluid or trying to excise and oversew a portion of the redundant wall. On rare occasion, when we are unable to find sperm in the vasal fluid or epididymal tubules, we may find many motile sperm in the epididymal cyst or cysts which may be a source of bankable sperm for future IVF/ICSI. More often, though, we do not find any sperm in the fluid within these cysts.

Discrepant Vasal Lumens

The vasal lumen in the abdominal vas is most often small and not dilated. The vasal lumen in the testicular vas can vary widely in size from quite small to very dilated as a result of distention from the buildup of vasal fluid under a head of pressure. In some men, the discrepancy can be dramatic (Fig. 8.4). A significant discrepancy in lumen size provides a technical challenge to approximate the lumen to lumen without gaps or overlap. The primary challenge with a significantly increased testicular lumen size is how to avoid gaps in between mucosal-to-mucosal approximation sutures where sperm and fluid can leak leading to subsequent anastomotic scarring. When there is significant dilation of the abdominal vas, I have found that the placement of an additional one to two mucosal sutures will reduce these gaps. Though I usually place six mucosal 10-0 nylon, sutures, with dramatically discrepant lumens, I often place seven or eight mucosal sutures. Of course, the downside to adding sutures is that we don't want to place too many sutures in the normal nondilated abdominal vas because of concerns over ischemic changes from compromise of the blood flow into the tissues. I have found that it helps to take a larger mucosal "bite" in the testicular lumen to help overcome any gaps during the anastomosis. The presence of a sperm granuloma usually is associated with a small, nondilated testicular vasal lumen small, similar in size to the abdominal vas.

Calcifications in the Vas

On rare occasions, you may unexpectedly encounter very dense calcifications scattered within the muscularis of the vas. None of the patients where we have found these scattered calcifications had any known explanations such as diabetes or any systemic illness nor any history of vasal infection or scrotal trauma. The challenges

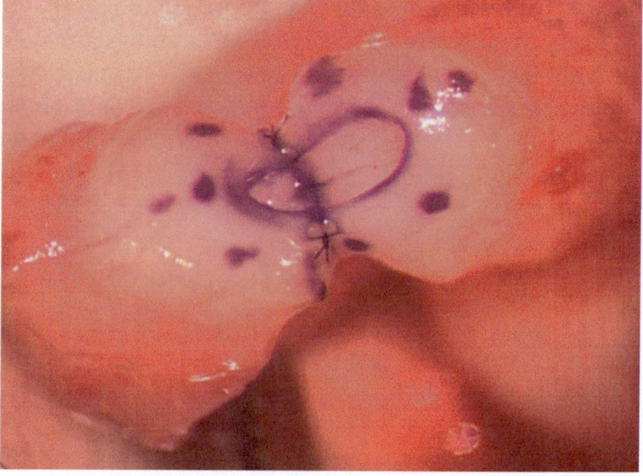

Fig. 8.4 Significantly dilated testicular vasal lumen. (Photo Credit: Sheldon Marks)

with these vasal calcifications are multiple. First, because of the inability to cut through the calcification with a microblade, it is difficult to transect the vas and obtain a clean face of healthy tissue. This forces the surgeon to have to move up the vas to find a segment of vas where there are no calcifications. Second, any attempted transection of the vas when encountering calcification instantly dulls the blade and leaves an irregular, partially calcified vasal face forcing a recut with a new blade. Most importantly, it is impossible to place microsutures through these calcified portions. Needles cannot be passed through the calcifications, so there are concerns about a watertight repair and that the tissues cannot heal together if you are unable to approximate healthy vas to healthy vas. When we have encountered unexpected vasal calcifications, we ask the patient to follow up with his primary care doctor for further evaluation and testing to look for a systemic illness that could explain the findings in the absence of any trauma, prior surgery, or infections.

Missing Vas and/or Portions of Epididymis

The absence of portions of the vas and/or epididymis is most consistent with iatrogenic injury or concerns over CBAVD (congenital bilateral absence of the vas deferens). At this point, if the reversal cannot be performed on this or the contralateral side, with no acceptable epididymal tubules above the gap, then we proceed with sperm retrieval. Afterward, we then review with the patient and his partner our concerns and the need for further genetic testing [3, 4].

Vasoepididymostomy Specific Dilemmas and Challenges

Some of the challenges and dilemmas seen with a VV can also apply to a VE, such as encountering a pouchy abdominal mucosa, calcifications in the vas, or lengthy vasal gap. There are predicaments we often find when performing a vasoepididymostomy that can make an already technically challenging procedure even more demanding.

No Fluid in the Epididymal Tubule

There are instances when you will open an epididymal tubule and find no visible fluid. This can resolve as fluid may begin to flow with time and gentle epididymal massage to milk the epididymal fluid toward the open tubule. If no fluid is seen, put a tiny drop of LR, NS, or HTF on the end of a sterile glass slide, and dab the drop on the glass slide onto the open defect as sometimes sperm can still be found microscopically. If no sperm are seen and no fluid noted, then you may try to very gently instill irrigant via a 24-gauge angiocath to see if perhaps you can pick up some sperm that might then be seen. If there is still no epididymal fluid, then you may need to abort that tubule and repeat the process opening up a new tubule higher along the epididymis. When doing so, it may help to look for any visible change in the color or appearance of the intratubular fluid for your new target tubule.

No Sperm or Sperm Parts in the Epididymal Fluid

If you are unable to find sperm or parts in epididymal fluid, then there are two explanations. One is that there is no sperm production from suppression or spermatogenic arrest. The other scenario is that you are below the level of epididymal obstruction and that the sperm are present though higher up in the epididymis. We regularly have encountered this situation when we were forced to create several epididymal windows to ultimately find a tubule with sperm, sometimes surprisingly high in the epididymis. There are times when the only sperm you find will be in the efferent ducts from a presumed high blowout with obstruction.

Vascular Surface of Epididymal Tunica

It can be frustrating when the tunica overlying the epididymal tubules is densely covered with blood vessels. The challenge is to examine the epididymis carefully under the microscope to find an avascular window where you can access an underlying tubule. There may be times when you have to use microbipolar to address blood vessels to make it possible to tease out and open an underlying tubule for the anastomosis.

Scarring with Thickened Epididymal Tunic

Dense scarring covering the epididymis makes visualization of the underlying tubules very difficult. Whether from prior surgery, infection, trauma, or unknown cause, it is especially challenging when you encounter overlying dense scar. This can be from the tunica vaginalis scarred down to the tunica albuginea, or it may be thick, dense scar overlying the epididymis. This can make identification of a tubule and subsequent preparation and vasoepididymostomy difficult. We then infiltrate the tissue with local anesthetic to separate the tissues and use low-power cautery or sharp dissection with microscissors to gently tease the scar off of the epididymis overlying the point when you anticipate performing the repair. This may then expose the tubules though with no overlying tunica to secure the abdominal vasal muscularis or adventitia. You will then need to improvise with sutures to whatever tissues you can find to secure and position the vas for the intussusception. There are instances when the tunica is thickened and not the expected thin, translucent covering over the epididymal tubules. This can make seeing and selecting the tubule difficult. If you encounter this dilemma, then in my experience, I choose a level where I anticipate I will find good epididymal tubules with sperm and blindly superficially score the thickened overlying tunica and then delicately separate and divide the tissues down with the microscissors until the tubules become visible.

Tiny, Flat, Nondilated Epididymal Tubules

You may encounter vasal fluid findings that support that an epididymal blowout occurred on one side, yet when you examine the epididymal tubules, you discover that they are flat, nondilated, and barely visible, if at all. This raise concerns that the patient may be suppressed or perhaps that he just has flat, minimally visible tubules. In my experience, we have found that these tubules can still have good sperm counts and motility. It is just that the finer, smaller-caliber tubules are usually more challenging to isolate and then to use for the intussusception vasoepididymostomy.

Maneuvers When There Is a Lengthy Gap

The goal is to have enough vasal length with epididymal positioning so that the vasoepididymostomy is not on any tension. First try and free up the abdominal vas from surrounding peri-vasal and cord attachments. This can often provide some additional length to bridge the gap, though in my experience usually not a significant amount. If this is insufficient, another trick is to incise the tunica between the distal epididymis and tunica albuginea of the bottom of the testicle. This should be done over the tunica of the testicle, away from the epididymis and under direct vison to avoid injury to underlying blood vessels. Most often this technique provides enough additional length to release the tethering as the tail of the epididymis is drawn up superiorly from the testicle (Fig. 8.5) [5].

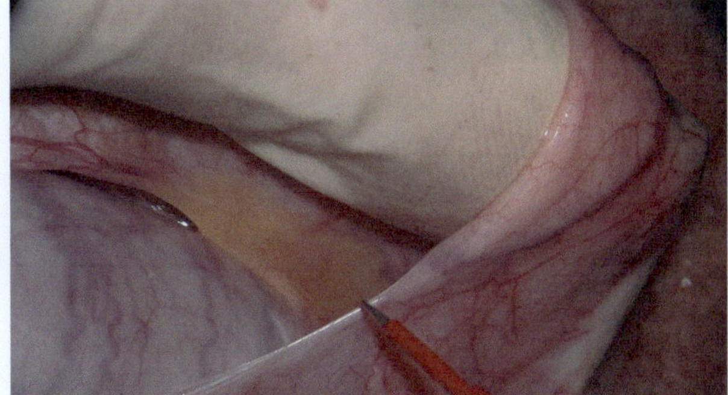

Fig. 8.5 Incision of the tunica between the distal epididymis and tunica albuginea of the bottom of the testicle to provide additional length to bring the tail of the epididymis superiorly for a vasoepididymostomy. (Photo Credit: Sheldon Marks)

References

1. Patel SR, Sigman M. Comparison of outcomes of vasovasostomy performed in the convoluted and straight vas deferens. J Urol. 2008;179:256–9.
2. Sandlow JI, Kolettis PN. Vasovasostomy in the convoluted vas deferens: indications and outcomes. J Urol. 2005;173:540–2.
3. Flannigan R, Schlegel PN. Genetic diagnostics of male infertility in clinical practice. Best Pract Res Clin Obstet Gynaecol. 2017 Oct;44:26–37.
4. de Souza DAS, Faucz FR, Pereira-Ferrari L, Sotomaior VS, Raskin S. Congenital bilateral absence of the vas deferens as an atypical form of cystic fibrosis: reproductive implications and genetic counseling. Andrology. 2018 Jan;6(1):127–35.
5. Chan PT. The evolution and refinement of vasoepididymostomy techniques. Asian J Androl. 2013;15:49–55. Asian J Androl 2016 Jan-Feb; 18(1): 129–133.

Chapter 9
Andrology Care

Andrology Services in a Reversal Practice

Many reversal doctors perform their own intraoperative vasal fluid analysis with an adjacent, tabletop lab microscope, while others may deliver the glass slides with the vasal fluid to a pathologist at a nearby lab or facility. This can be time-consuming, adding delays in decision-making and so operative time. If sperm banking is needed, surgeons can arrange for an outside lab to be present at the time of the reversal, or the doctor can have the sperm transported to a lab for cryopreservation. We have found that having our own in-house, full-time andrologist overcomes all of these hurdles and significantly reduces surgical time and improves the outcomes and quality of intraop and postop care for our reversal patients. Plus, having an andrologist as part of the reversal team provides the option to perform an intraoperative diagnostic TESE or bank sperm at any time during or after the reversal.

Benefits of Intraoperative Andrology Skills

There are two ways to analyze the vasal fluid real time to assess whether the system is open and a vasovasostomy is indicated or if there is no sperm which may be suggestive of deeper epididymal obstruction and so a VE is indicated. One is to do it yourself and the other is to delegate this task to an andrologist. Most doctors simply look through a high-quality, high-power (100X) lab microscope setup in the OR to analyze the vasal fluid. The advantage to this approach is that it is quick, provides direct visualization for the doctor which is important with indeterminate fluid, and does not require any additional staffing. The disadvantage to the surgeon alone looking at the slide is that if sperm are not seen right away, it can be time-consuming for the doctor to slowly scan the slide hunting for rare sperm or sperm parts, always

© Springer Nature Switzerland AG 2019

S. H. F. Marks, *Vasectomy Reversal*,

https://doi.org/10.1007/978-3-030-00455-2_9

with a chance that sperm will be present but not seen, and so the doctor may incorrectly assume that the lack of visible sperm suggests deeper epididymal blockage and perform the more complicated VE with a lower likelihood of success.

Because we have a full-time andrologist at our reversal center, when we hand off the slides, he immediately begins scanning and looking for sperm while we are able to continue the surgery. In our practice, on a regular basis, the andrologist has been able to perform a more comprehensive microscopic analysis of the fluid and find rare and even motile sperm when none were seen on the surgeon's own review of the slide. This obviously allowed us to perform a vasovasostomy with much higher and quicker success that if we had relied on the surgeon's inability to see any sperm and so defaulted to a VE, incorrectly assuming that no sperm were present in the vasal fluid. In order to see what the andrologist is visualizing on his lab scope, we have monitors in the OR that allows the surgeon to see the best-quality sperm and decide if a VV or VE is indicated [1–5]. Having a highly skilled and trained andrologist enables the surgeon to perform a VV with higher success, while allowing the surgical team to continue with the reversal while the andrologist is actively looking for sperm. This is much more time efficient and provides for better results for the patients.

Role of an Andrologist with TESE

An andrologist has been essential at times when we discover intraoperatively that we need to perform a real-time diagnostic TESE or perform testicular sperm extraction for cryopreservation. This can be necessary and valuable when no sperm are seen in the epididymal fluid. This may be an issue if there are concerns over sperm suppression from prior or covert continued testosterone therapy or even unsuspected compromised spermatogenesis from any number of causes or obstruction at the level of the efferent ducts. Of course, the technique of teasing apart the seminiferous tubules and then examining the tissue for sperm is tedious and time-consuming. Sometimes sperm are seen in good numbers, and so results can be relayed to the surgeon quickly to help in decision-making. There are other instances where no sperm are seen initially, and more tissue or time is needed for a comprehensive review.

Andrology Services After the Reversal

We have discovered that much of the success of a reversal comes from close aftercare. Whether performing semen analyses or interpreting outside lab results, the in-house andrologist significantly improves patient care and reduces time demands on the surgeon. Many andrologists, working closely with the urologist, play a critical role in the interpretation of lab reports and recommendations for care of the patient's serial post-reversal semen analyses. Our andrologist is able to review and interpret reports, compare to past levels, and work with the doctor to formulate a treatment plan, if needed, for management of suboptimal or decreasing semen parameters. Quite often patients will talk with our andrologist with their questions about the role of nutrition, diet, supplements, the impact of their occupation and lifestyle, as well as options to optimize male and female fertility.

Banking, Intraop or Delayed

During the reversal is probably the best and easiest time to perform sperm retrieval for cryopreservation and banking. If there is adequate fluid volume, sperm counts and motility, then the vasal or epididymal fluid can be aspirated in sperm wash media (HTF) and delivered to your andrologist for cryopreservation should ART be required in the future. Even though the chances that the patient will require the banked sperm in the future are low, many patients prefer to have sperm frozen, if given the option [6–8]. Those rare patients that did need banked sperm were grateful for having the option for cryopreservation years before. Having the andrologist there is helpful to determine real time if the specimen delivered is adequate for banking or if additional vasal or epididymal fluid or if more testicular tissue is required.

Sperm Disposition if Death

Anytime that sperm cryopreservation is performed and banked at the time of the reversal, it is important when consenting for the sperm banking that you also address the disposition and ownership of the frozen sperm in the case of the patient's future death. It is also wise to discuss and consent whether or not the patient gives his permission to his partner to use the sperm post-mortem for fathering of future children.

References

1. Kolettis PN, Burns JR, Nangia AK, Sandlow JI. Outcomes for vasovasostomy performed when only sperm parts are present in the vasal fluid. J Androl. 2006;27:565–7.
2. Kolettis PN, D'Amico AM, Box L, et al. Outcomes for vasovasostomy with bilateral intravasal azoospermia. J Androl. 2003;24:22–4.
3. Scovell JM, Mata DA, Ramasamy R, et al. Association between the presence of sperm in the vasal fluid during vasectomy reversal and postoperative patency: a systematic review and meta-analysis. Urology. 2015;85:809–13.
4. Smith RP, Khanna A, Kovac JR, et al. The significance of sperm heads and tails within the vasal fluid during vasectomy reversal. Indian J Urol. 2014;30:164–8.

5. Ramasamy R, Mata DA, Jain L, Perkins AR, Marks SH, Lipshultz LI. Microscopic visualization of intravasal spermatozoa is positively associated with patency after bilateral microsurgical vasovasostomy. Andrology. 2015;3(3):532–5.
6. Glazier DB, Marmar JL, Mayer E, Gibbs M, Corson SL. The fate of cryopreserved sperm acquired during vasectomy reversals. J Urol. 1999;161:463–6.
7. Boyle KE, Thomas AJ Jr, Marmar JL, Hirshberg S, Belker AM, Jarow JP. Sperm harvesting and cryopreservation during vasectomy reversal is not cost effective. Fertil Steril. 2006;85:961–4.
8. Schrepferman CG, Carson MR, Sparks AE, Sandlow JI. Need for sperm retrieval and cryopreservation at vasectomy reversal. J Urol. 2001;166:1787–9.

Chapter 10
Post-reversal Management and Care

Post-reversal discharge instructions can be just as important to the uneventful recovery and outcome of your patient's reversal as the technical aspects of the vasectomy reversal itself. Because couples have invested so much emotionally and financially into the results of the reversal, providing detailed patient educational materials is critical to your patient's care so that they know what to do and, more importantly, what not to do. Even with clear instructions, many men will still not follow your guidelines. This is why we provide not only the instructions or precautions but also the rationale for that guideline. We also understand that the brief postoperative conversation with the patient and his partner is quickly forgotten, and so a customized booklet of care is sent home with each patient. The goal is to empower the patient to understand acceptable and recommended behaviors. With this knowledge, he and his partner can make wise choices after the reversal to avoid modifiable behaviors that may compromise the recovery and increase risks for risks and complications [1, 2].

Written and Verbal Discharge Instructions: What You Say Versus What They Remember

When considering thepost-reversal instructions that you give to your patients, it is not what you say but what they remember. This is why it is so important to provide detailed written instructions [3]. In a normal situation, it is impossible for a nonmedical person to be able to recall all the findings, postop care, and instructions for today, tomorrow, next week, and next month. Add to this the emotional stress of surgery and the normal amnesic impact of the sedatives, and you can almost guarantee that most of what you or others told the patient will not be remembered or will be recalled incorrectly. We limit our review to key concepts and limited instructions of important points of his aftercare with the patient and his partner and

© Springer Nature Switzerland AG 2019

S. H. F. Marks, *Vasectomy Reversal*,

https://doi.org/10.1007/978-3-030-00455-2_10

then accompany those verbal instructions with customized written detailed instructions to include the rationale behind those instructions. Having this reference empowers the patient and his partner to be better team players in their care.

Immediate Recovery and Care

The initial care of your reversal patient can impact on how comfortable they are as well as the ultimate outcomes. In addition to the standard postanesthesia and postop care and instructions, we include a number of reversal specific instructions. Standard postop generic instructions alone from the facility or center are inadequate. It is also important to address patient-specific issues such as return to work, hobbies, and sports.

Ice

Our patients are instructed to apply ice over the scrotum, 30 min on and 10 min off, for the first 48–72 h. We emphasize that the ice should be applied outside the underwear, never directly against the skin, nor should it be placed over multiple layers of thick insulating clothing or blankets. Ideally, a thin layer of clothing such as underwear should protect the skin from the ice. The ice can be discontinued when the patient is sleeping at night, to be restarted in the morning.

Athletic Supporter

We have found that the patients feel better when they wear an athletic supporter or bicycle/compression shorts over their underwear for the first 2 weeks, as tolerated. This helps to minimize testicular movement and coincidentally provides a place to hold the ice packs in position over the scrotum.

Restrictions on Activity

Patients are asked to stay off their feet after surgery for the first 48–72 h and then avoid any prolonged standing, squatting, heavy lifting, or straining for the first 2 weeks to prevent any bleeding or pain. Any personal, sports, or occupational activities should be addressed specifically. In my experience, if you don't talk about returning to normal activities or a topic of concern, then they will assume that it is okay to begin training for an upcoming triathlon or sky diving 5 days post-reversal. Despite sharing our concerns and instructions, we have had patients resume riding their road bike 60–100 miles a day just 3 days post-reversal, and another went back to professional rodeo bull riding 2 weeks after his surgery.

Incisional Care

Each patient is given a detailed information sheet outlining incisional care and expectations for intermittent bleeding with normal healing scenarios as well as warning signs for possible infection.

Discharge Medications

This is a topic where you must be very clear about what the patient can and cannot take and when they can be resumed, specifically addressing the dose and regimens of every medication that you prescribe. We discharge the patient with a detailed list of side effects and potential risks with every prescribed medication. We emphasize that whether prescription or over-the-counter, many medications and supplements can negatively interact with other medications, increase risks for bleeding, or can be sperm toxic so it is important to work with our office before they take any product.

Resumption of Normal Medications and Supplements

Depending on the medication or supplement, some are restarted immediately after the surgery without a break, to continue on their regular pre-reversal dose and regimen. Others may be resumed after a day or two delay or longer, again medication and patient specific. Many patients will almost immediately start taking a variety of healing, anti-inflammatory supplements, so it is important to ask about these specifically with your patients.

Antiplatelet or Blood Thinners

Because some of the patients have a medical reason to be on these medications, whether an over-the-counter aspirin or more powerful blood thinners, we coordinate with their doctor when these are to be restarted. Some have to be restarted right away, while others can be delayed days to a week or more post-reversal.

Antibiotics Post-reversal

The use of post-reversal prophylactic antibiotics varies widely among experts. Some strictly follow the guidelines and do not prescribe any postop antibiotics, while others may prescribe a few doses. We use one dose of cephazolin (Kefzol) preoperatively and then continue oral cephalexin (Keflex) for a few doses post-reversal [4].

Anti-inflammatory Medications

If the patient was found to have a sperm granuloma, if there was extensive, dense peri-vasal scarring or after a redo salvage reversal with concerns for excessive inflammation, we often prescribe a tapering course of steroids, either prednisone or methylprednisolone to be followed by NSAIDs for a full 6-week course. We prefer the use of celecoxib or meloxicam as neither is associated with the compromise of platelet function and so should not increase risks for postop bleeding [5, 6].

Pain Medications

Most of our reversal patients rarely need to take even a single acetaminophen, but just in case of moderate discomfort, we provide several regular strength tablets in their discharge medications. We include a review of the indications, precautions, side effects, and warnings of these medications in each patient's discharge material [7]. We have found that with meticulous surgery and sensible use of local anesthetics, it is rare for reversal patients to need any narcotics postoperatively.

Delayed Care, Precautions, and Restrictions

Most men can resume their normal activities and work at about 10–14 days after the reversal, though for those with exceptionally physical occupations or hobbies such as weight lifting, we encourage that they avoid the most strenuous core activities for a full 3–4 weeks. Though they may feel fine and all "healed," we explain that the tissues are still in the very early phases of healing and traumatic activities can cause significant swelling, possible bleeding, and pain. We ask our patients to avoid strenuous activity and aggressive core exercises such as squats, crunches, and leg presses for 4–6 weeks. Likewise, we ask that our patients avoid activities that are potentially traumatic to freshly healing repair such as long-distance road bike riding, horseback riding, or similar behaviors. If they have any specific strenuous behavior with their work, sports, or hobbies, then it is best to provide very specific guidelines and precautions. We discuss the importance of avoiding excessive heat to the scrotum indefinitely as long as they are trying to conceive [8].

Resuming Sexual Activity

We recommend that our patients abstain from ejaculation and sexual activity for 14 days after a vasovasostomy or vasoepididymostomy. There are concerns that a longer period of abstinence might increase the risks for progression of inflammation and obstruction of the fresh anastomosis. In addition, many couples have admitted that at about 14 days they are going to begin sexual activity anyway, even if we ask for longer interval of abstinence.

Frequency of Ejaculation

After the reversal we do encourage regular ejaculation, every 24–48 h around the time of ovulation. We explain the issues and how too frequent an ejaculation or too infrequent can impact on fertility.

Compliance with Discharge Instructions

We continue to be surprised how often men will not follow these post-reversal instructions, often restarting aggressive sports or physical activities right after surgery, taking a variety of herbs and supplements without checking with our office, or just stopping the ice after the first postop night. Some men are compliant, while many others have told us that since they felt fine, they just assumed it was okay to begin activities much earlier than clearly addressed in the discharge instructions. We believe that our post-reversal discharge educational materials and regular postop follow-up by our office help to reduce noncompliance [9, 10].

Follow-Up Semen Analyses

We encourage frequent and regular monitoring of the semen analyses to follow sperm counts closely, starting at 4 weeks and continuing every 4 weeks until stable and acceptable results. Close monitoring of the counts will help us to identify trends early on and so allow for the opportunity for pharmacologic intervention during that window of opportunity if we see suboptimal counts or decreasing counts, suggestive of excessive intraluminal inflammation and progressive anastomotic scarring.

We point out to our patients that a semen analysis is a valuable tool to monitor the results of the reversal. We want our patients to understand that a semen analysis is a measure of both sperm production and delivery and not a good measure of fertility. Our office emphasizes that anything that can impact on sperm production and quality can hurt or help the numbers just as scarring or inflammation can hurt the flow of sperm through the vas connection.

Compliance with Post-reversal Semen Analysis

We have found that patient compliance for post-reversal semen analysis testing, in general, is poor for most men after their reversal. Many couples incorrectly assume that they will have great results and that semen analyses are an unnecessary nuisance. Even though we explain how important follow-up semen analysis testing is to achieve the best results, many men often do not check a sperm count for months, if at all. Some mistakenly believe that they should try to conceive, and if nothing happened in 6–12 months, then they will check a sperm count. Reasons men often provide to not check a semen analysis as requested include that they were too busy, they simply forgot, or testing was inconvenient or expensive. In our own review of 389 patients, we found that 15% were not compliant with providing specimens for semen analysis at recommended intervals [11]. The battle with testing is between obtaining real-time actionable information, so we can intervene with anti-inflammatory medications as the counts are dropping, and patient inconvenience or cost. If the patient is asked to provide a semen analysis too often, then they will often stop providing specimens after just a few. If you have too long of an interval between testing, then you lose that window of opportunity when you are best able to treat early inflammatory obstruction and restore sperm counts back to target levels.

References

1. Rossi BV, Abusief M, Missmer SA. Modifiable risk factors and infertility: what are the connections? Am J Lifestyle Med. 2014;10(4):220–31.
2. Sharma R, Biedenharn KR, Fedor JM, Argawal A. Lifestyle factors and reproductive health: taking control of your fertility. Reprod Biol Endocrinol. 2013;11:66.
3. Davies N, Papa N, Ischia J, Bolton D, Lawrentschuk N. Consistency of written post-operative patient information for common urological procedures. ANZ J Surg. 2015;85(12):941–5.
4. Wolf JS Jr, Bennett CJ, Dmochowski RR, Hollenbeck BK, Pearle MS, Schaeffer AJ, Urologic Surgery Antimicrobial Prophylaxis Best Practice Policy Panel. Best practice policy statement on urologic surgery antimicrobial prophylaxis. J Urol. 2008;179(4):1379–90.

5. Teerawattananon C, Tantayakom P, Suwanawiboon B, Katchamart W. Risk of perioperative bleeding related to highly selective cyclooxygenase-2 inhibitors: a systematic review and meta-analysis. Semin Arthritis Rheum. 2017;46(4):520–8.
6. Perkins A, Marks MB, Peter Burrows PJ, Marks SF. Anti-inflammatory treatment for asthenozoospermia following microsurgical vasectomy reversal. Presented at American Society of Andrology 38th Annual Meeting, San Antonio, Texas: April 13–17, 2013.
7. Fujii MH, Hodges AC, Russell RL, Roensch K, Beynnon B, Ahern TP, Holoch P, Moore JS, Ames SE, MacLean CD. Post-discharge opioid prescribing and use after common surgical procedures. J Am Coll Surg. 2018. pii: S1072-7515(18)30154-6; https://doi.org/10.1016/j.jamcollsurg.2018.01.058.
8. Rao M, Zhao XL, Yang J, Hu SF, Lei H, Xia W, Zhu CH. Effect of transient scrotal hyperthermia on sperm parameters, seminal plasma biochemical markers, and oxidative stress in men. Asian J Androl. 2015;17(4):668–75.
9. Maatman TJ, Aldrin L, Carothers GG. Patient noncompliance after vasectomy. Fertil Steril. 1997;68:552–5.
10. Sheynkin Y, Mishail A, Vemulapalli P, Lee J, Ahn H, Schulsinger D. Sociodemographic predictors of postvasectomy noncompliance. Contraception. 2009;80:566–8.
11. Murphy R, Perkins A, Marks MB, Burrows PJ, Marks SF. Post vasectomy reversal semen analysis compliancy. Androl. 2012;33(Suppl 2):42.

Chapter 11
Complications of Vasectomy Reversals

Complications of a vasectomy reversal are the same as any potential risks and complications after a vasectomy or any other scrotal/testicular surgery. In skilled and experienced hands, these complications are rare but can still happen. If you have not had one of these complications, it is probably because you have not performed enough reversals. In our experience, these risks and complication occur less often with a reversal than a vasectomy, perhaps because the entire reversal is performed microsurgically under direct vison. A review of these and other reversal specific and general potential risks and complications should be reviewed at the time of your preoperative informed consent. By including the patient in the discussion of these risks, then if signs or symptoms of any problems appear, he is more likely to initiate early intervention and so have better outcomes. These risks are more likely when the patient has had previous successful or unsuccessful reconstruction attempts, other scrotal/testicular/inguinal surgeries, or when more aggressive surgery is required to isolate the vas, epididymis, or testicle from extensive scar or to free up and mobilize the abdominal vas or the epididymis. These prior surgeries and procedures can result in extensive scarring and disruption of normal vascular supply and tissue planes, which make an already challenging surgery even more difficult. Other than failure of the reversal, which is addressed below, here are some of the most common complications after a reversal.

Bleeding, Immediate and Delayed

Bleeding can occur with any surgery, immediately after the procedure or days to weeks later. Though we expect to see some mild bruising and swelling, significant and rapid development of an expanding ecchymosis and dramatic swelling with pain is evidence of post-reversal bleeding and hematoma formation. If the bleed and hematoma are large enough or developing rapidly, the pain can be severe and prolonged. Though some can be managed conservatively, others may require surgical

© Springer Nature Switzerland AG 2019

S. H. F. Marks, *Vasectomy Reversal*,

https://doi.org/10.1007/978-3-030-00455-2_11

exploration to identify the bleeding site and remove any clot. It is rare to find the source of any bleeding among the disrupted bloody tissues, where it can seem that all the tissues are raw and oozing blood. Examination will confirm the presumptive diagnosis of an acute bleed and hematoma. For delayed pain with more insidious, chronic swelling, a testicular ultrasound can better define the anatomy and the presence of a hematoma or possible testicular atrophy [1].

Scrotal Drains

If you have concerns during the reversal over the development of a scrotal hematoma from continued oozing of blood from extensive raw surfaces, then an intrascrotal drain or drains can be placed and left in either or both sides overnight or longer as needed. In the past when we left in a drain, we preferred to use a 1/4 inch latex Penrose drain. However, to keep our OR latex free, in those rare situations where a drain is needed, we have switched over to use a firmer and so less desirable Silastic product. The drain or drains are then placed deep in the hemiscrotal compartments and brought out through the inferior aspect of the incision and then secured with a sterile safety pin to the overlying gauze. The attached gauze and drains are then easily removed with firm and steady traction the next morning after the reversal. When we do use two drains, we cut the left drain at an angle and know that the right drain is cut at a right angle.

Infection

Infections are very rare after vasectomy reversal when you follow appropriate standards and meticulous technique for care and handling of tissues. The routine use of pre- and post-reversal antibiotics remains controversial [2]. Most experts use broad-spectrum intravenous cephalosporin at the time of the reversal and for a few oral doses after. We do review with the patient early warning signs and symptoms of a possible infection with instructions to contact us immediately. More often than not, the patients will mistakenly think that signs of normal postop inflammation are a sign of infection. Examination and treatment with broad-spectrum antibiotics are indicated if there are any concerns.

Hydrocele

A reactive hydrocele after a vasectomy reversal is rarely seen, but if it occurs, it is most often unilateral and not significant in size. If present, it usually causes patient concern. We counsel our patients that most often, a reactive hydrocele will resolve with time and conservative management. Rarely will a hydrocele require intervention.

Testicular Atrophy

Testicular atrophy, acute and delayed, can result from compromise of the testicular blood supply during or after a vasectomy reversal. Though extremely rare, atrophy can occur most often following a challenging redo reversal, with other prior testicular/scrotal surgeries/trauma, or from development of a postop cord hematoma with a form of a localized spermatic cord compartment syndrome. Testicular atrophy can be acute, occurring shortly after the reversal, or delayed, developing weeks to months later. Testicular atrophy may initially present as significant and progressive testicular swelling and pain beyond what you would normally expect and then a slow reduction in testicular size over months. Delayed testicular atrophy may present with a slow decrease in the size of the testicle, with or without pain. A color flow Doppler is a valuable tool to help identify if there are any ischemic changes or reduced blood flow. If there are early acute changes associated with a spermatic cord hematoma, then surgical decompression may be indicated.

Testicular Pain

Pain after a vasectomy reversal, similar to post-vasectomy pain syndrome (PVPS), is seen very rarely. This post-reversal pain could be as a result of extreme peri-vasal inflammation, perhaps as a result of a sperm leak at the anastomotic site with a subsequent inflammatory sperm granuloma, possibly a small peri-vasal hematoma, possibly higher cord issues such as peri-vasal inflammation and scarring from a hernia or herniorrhaphy mesh, or perhaps genetically mediated Wallerian degeneration. As we know with PVPS patients, there is rarely an obvious etiology, and so treatments are directed at controlling the pain and symptoms. This is rare as the majority of men who have a vasectomy reversal for the treatment of severe PVPS do very well with significant or complete resolution of their pain [3–9].

References

1. Johnson D, Sandlow JI. Vasectomy: tips and tricks. Transl Androl Urol. 2017;6(4):704–9.
2. Wolf JS Jr, Bennett CJ, Dmochowski RR, Hollenbeck BK, Pearle MS, Schaeffer AJ, Urologic Surgery Antimicrobial Prophylaxis Best Practice Policy Panel. Best practice policy statement on urologic surgery antimicrobial prophylaxis. J Urol. 2008;179(4):1379–90.
3. Leslie TA, Illing RO, Cranston DW, et al. The incidence of chronic scrotal pain after vasectomy: a prospective audit. BJU Int. 2007;100:1330–3.
4. Tandon S, Sabanegh E Jr. Chronic pain after vasectomy: a diagnostic and treatment dilemma. BJU Int. 2008;102:166–9.
5. Myers SA, Mershon CE, Fuchs EF. Vasectomy reversal for treatment of the post-vasectomy pain syndrome. J Urol. 1997;157:518–20.

6. Lee JY, Chang JS, Lee SH, Ham WS, Cho HJ, Yoo TK, Lee KS, Kim TH, Moon HS, Choi HY, Lee SW. Efficacy of vasectomy reversal according to patency for the surgical treatment of postvasectomy pain syndrome. Int J Impot Res. 2012;24(5):202–5.
7. Sinha V, Ramasamy R. Post-vasectomy pain syndrome: diagnosis, management and treatment options. Transl Androl Urol. 2017;6(Suppl 1):S44–7.
8. Smith-Harrison LI, Smith RP. Vasectomy reversal for post-vasectomy pain syndrome. Transl Androl Urol. 2017;6(Suppl 1):S10–3.
9. Schmidt SS. Spermatic granuloma: an often painful lesion. Fertil Steril. 1979;31(2):178–81.

Chapter 12
Sperm Kinetics After VV or VE and Reversal Failure

After a bilateral vasovasostomy, most patients can expect to see sperm on the first semen analyses at 30 days, with counts and motility continuing to improve over several consecutive months. The better the quality of the sperm seen in the vasal fluid predicts for earlier and better outcomes in most men. Of course, as it takes 74–90 days to make a sperm, so it may be a few months until optimal sperm parameters in an obstructed system are achieved. The presence of a sperm granuloma on one or both sides most often is associated with an excellent and quick return of good sperm parameters, though always with the concern for persistent inflammation leading to delayed anastomotic failure. After a vasoepididymostomy, the return of sperm to the ejaculate can be quite variable and unpredictable, with sperm seen anytime from the first semen analysis at 4 weeks up to 6–12 months or more [1–3]. The best scenarios are when the sperm returns to the counts sooner rather than later, usually by 4–6 months. There are men who will see sperm return to the ejaculate even 18–36 months or longer. It is important to counsel your patients about this widely variable and unpredictable return of sperm, as the initial zero sperm counts are usually very frustrating and disappointing for couples. Even with this information, many couples still expect almost immediate results and will stop checking semen analyses after several months, becoming discouraged and incorrectly assuming that an azoospermic semen analysis means the reversal was a failure. Because there is always a chance for future anastomotic stricturing progressing to obstruction with subsequent azoospermia, we always recommend that patients who have good counts with high motility should cryopreserve sperm for future IUI or IVF/ICSI, just in case.

© Springer Nature Switzerland AG 2019
S. H. F. Marks, *Vasectomy Reversal*,
https://doi.org/10.1007/978-3-030-00455-2_12

Management of Suboptimal or Decreasing Counts/Motility Post-reversal

There are several common scenarios we can see after a reversal for low numbers or a drop in the sperm parameters. One is that the post-reversal semen analyses remain azoospermic or with a very poor concentration or motility over several lab tests. The other is that the sperm counts normalize for a period of time and then on subsequent follow-up semen analyses the concentration and/or motility drops significantly and can even become azoospermic. The persistence of poor counts or dropping sperm parameters suggests that you did the correct procedure and that there is either significant inflammation or that there is suppressed sperm production. In both of these scenarios, because we want to intervene as soon as possible, we would assume that there is excessive inflammation and treat the patient with a course of anti-inflammatory medications such as a tapering course of prednisone or methylprednisolone to be followed by NSAIDs or NSAIDs alone [4]. Most often, if the low counts are a result of anastomotic inflammation, then they usually increase over the next semen analysis or two. We also talk with the patient trying to identify any possible explanations for sperm suppression, either before and/or after the reversal. On occasion the patient will admit to restarting testosterone therapy, a high fever or illness after the reversal, or initiating a new medication or lifestyle behavior that may be the cause of the azoospermia or low counts. There have been patients with high counts of whole motile sperm in the vasal fluid with an uneventful vasovasostomy and yet they still present with azoospermia on their first and subsequent semen analyses, suggesting a rapid onset of obstructing inflammation and scarring. The concern with consistent azoospermia post-vasovasostomy with indeterminate vasal fluid findings that you may have performed the wrong procedure and that a vasoepididymostomy was indicated. Even with this, we still would try to identify any modifiable causes and treat accordingly.

Failure of the Vasectomy Reversal: VV and VE

Failure of a reversal means different things to the doctors and to your patients. For reversal surgeons, a successful reversal means that the patient achieved adequate motile sperm in the ejaculate after a vasectomy reversal. After all, that's the goal. Unlike IVF, we are not making the baby. A failure to reversal surgeons means that no or inadequate sperm are getting through the anastomosis. We understand that a reversal is still considered successful even if the patient achieves good sperm counts and motility, but the couple does not conceive. Just as frustrating is when the patient achieves excellent semen parameters but then develops subsequent anastomotic scarring over time leading to poor counts or even azoospermia. Sadly, many times we see issues with dropping sperm counts as a result of poor patient compliance obtaining follow-up semen analyses or taking prescribed medications. It is generally accepted that a reversal failure is the inability to see any sperm in the ejaculate by 6 months following a bilateral vasovasostomy. After a bilateral vasoepididymostomy, we declare the reversal a failure if no sperm are seen by 18 months. Of course, we have seen many men who open up with good sperm counts after 18–36 months following a bilateral vasoepididymostomy [5–8].

To patients, even if they achieve and maintain excellent normal sperm parameters and they are not pregnant, they will still call to find out why the reversal was "not a success." Even after you explain that technically we restored good sperm counts and motility to the semen, and that conception and pregnancy is a multifactorial male and female driven event, they often naturally still feel sad, frustrated, and discouraged. This is where regular, open communication and continuing patient education plays an important role to ensure that the patient and his partner have appropriate expectations. Our andrologist, the nurses, and doctors stay actively involved to work with couples if there are any issues or concerns. If the couple has been trying for some time with good sperm counts, then we suggest a referral to a reproductive endocrinologist to be sure that the female partner is fertile and can conceive.

Possible Causes of Reversal Failure

Some of the possible causes for failure of a VV or VE, in addition to incorrect intraoperative decision-making or poor microsurgical technique include:

1. Undetected proximal abdominal vasal obstruction.
2. Failure to recognize and bypass epididymal obstruction and so a VV performed when a VE was indicated.
3. Sutures are tied too loose, so sperm can leak with resultant inflammation and scar.
4. Sutures are tied too tight with subsequent ischemia in the enclosed tissues, inflammation, and scarring.
5. Vasal damage from excessive cautery or bipolar.
6. Traumatic technique for passing of the microneedles.
7. Incorrect microneedles or sutures.
8. Inadequate blood supply with ischemia of the tissues, possible atrophy of the vas and/or testicle.
9. Poor intraoperative hemostasis with peri-vasal or peri-anastomotic bleeding.
10. Incorrect epididymal tubule selection with higher epididymal obstruction.
11. Failure to postoperatively identify and treat signs of anastomotic inflammation or stricture development.
12. Lastly, even if the reversal is done correctly using state-of-the-art techniques with correct decision-making, the patient's own genetic response to the trauma of the surgery and healing can result in uncontrollable post-reversal scarring and failure. Sometimes we have seen obstruction right away, even before the first semen analysis. Most often anastomotic scarring and blockage occurs months later and can be can be rapid or slow.

When the patient has a significant drop in sperm parameters or become azoospermic, you should always consider overt and covert patient lifestyle choices, illicit drugs, unknown or new illness, or medications or supplements, most notably testosterone replacement. Sadly, we regularly encounter many men who do not admit to staying on testosterone therapy or restarting testosterone at some point after the reversal. If there are concerns, then checking hormone levels is reasonable. Also, some men may be started without your knowledge on gonadotoxic medications by their doctors or even over-the-counter supplements. It is important to ask your patients to let you know about any health issues or new medications they may be on after the reversal. Many times, the patient's physicians are unaware of the potential for sperm compromising impact of many of the medications they prescribe. Of course, a significant systemic or febrile illness can also compromise sperm parameters, so it's not always anastomotic inflammation.

Prevention of Anastomotic Scarring

The standard technical suggestions to minimize post-reversal scarring and obstruction are universal, whether performing a microsurgical vasectomy reversal or any surgery. These include attention to meticulous surgical technique, minimizing damage to and handling of delicate tissues, prevention of tissue desiccation, regular irrigation to eliminate debris and clot, appropriate techniques or passage of the needles and tying the sutures, avoidance of excessive cautery or bipolar near the vas and epididymis, as well as close monitoring of serial semen analyses. As addressed earlier, if we encounter excessive scarring or peri-vasal inflammation at the time of the reversal, such as with a sperm granuloma, then we often have the patient take a course of steroidal or nonsteroidal anti-inflammatory medications post-reversal.

References

1. Perkins A, Marks MB, Burrows PJ, Marks SF. Sperm kinetics following vasectomy reversal. American Society of Andrology, 37th Annual Meeting, Tucson, Arizona. April 21–24, 2012.
2. Yang G, Walsh TJ, Shefi S, Turek PJ. The kinetics of the return of motile sperm to the ejaculate after vasectomy reversal. J Urol. 2007;177(6):2272–6.
3. Matthews GJ, Schlegel PN, Goldstein M. Patency following microsurgical vasoepididymostomy and vasovasostomy: temporal considerations. J Urol. 1995;154:2070–3.
4. Perkins A, Marks MB, Burrows PJ, Marks SF. Anti-inflammatory treatment for asthenozoospermia following microsurgical vasectomy reversal. Poster at the American Society of Andrology, 38th Annual Meeting, San Antonio, Texas. April 13–17, 2013.
5. Royle MG, Hendry WF. Why does vasectomy reversal fail? Br J Urol. 1985;57(6):780–3.
6. Schiff J, Chan P, Li PS, Finkelberg S, Goldstein M. Outcome and late failures compared in 4 techniques of microsurgical vasoepididymostomy in 153 consecutive men. J Urol. 2005;174:651–5.
7. Carbone DJ Jr, Shah A, Thomas AJ Jr, Agarwal A. Partial obstruction, not antisperm antibodies, causing infertility after vasovasostomy. J Urol. 1998;159:827–30.
8. Silber SJ. Epididymal extravasation following vasectomy as a cause for failure of vasectomy reversal. Fertil Steril. 1979;31:309–15.

Chapter 13
Redo "Salvage" Vasectomy Reversal

Redo Salvage Vasectomy Reversals

If an initial reversal fails, then for selected patients a redo or salvage reversal may be a reasonable option if the patient understands the unique challenges and limitations, both with intraoperative decision-making and, technically, when attempting to reverse a failed first attempt. Success of redo reversals can be very high in skilled, experienced hands [1–5]. Redo reversals are more likely to be successful if there was a return of sperm into the ejaculate before becoming azoospermic. This delayed obstruction is most often consistent with development of a post-op anastomotic stricture rather than originally performing an incorrect procedure [6]. Of course, anyone that has performed redo reversals will tell you that redo salvage reversals are inherently more challenging and time-consuming. Though most of our redo reversal are from failed reversal attempts elsewhere, on occasion we have to perform a redo reversal of our own reversal. Almost always at the time of the surgery you will encounter significant, dense peri-vasal and even peri-testicular scarring. We often will find total obliteration of normal tissue planes, especially if there was reported post-reversal bleeding, infection, or an attempted VE with the first reversal attempt. As Dr. Harris Nagler reminded me many years ago, "redo reversals are never easy." Of course, there are other possible explanations for the patient's azoospermia, so it is important to address these such suppression of spermatogenesis by testosterone therapy. If there are any questions or concerns, it may be reasonable to obtain a panel of hormone levels prior to the redo reversal. We usually check an FSH, LH, testosterone, and estradiol as a baseline if we are uncertain if there might be other etiologies for the presumed failure of the first reversal.

© Springer Nature Switzerland AG 2019

S. H. F. Marks, *Vasectomy Reversal*,

https://doi.org/10.1007/978-3-030-00455-2_13

Success of a Redo Reversal

Redo reversals from first attempts elsewhere are a major part of any busy reversal experts practice. A review of our own results with hundreds of redo reversals showed that in 99% of patients, we can achieve a successful outcome, almost as good as if the redo had been the patient's first reversal attempt [7]. Many consider a redo reversal still more cost-effective for selected patients than moving directly to IVF with ICSI [8]. Of course, much will depend on your own experience and many patient/partner specific and prior redo issues [9]. When we counsel prospective patients about a redo reversal, we are very clear that whatever led to the failure of the first attempt may still be at play, and so we discuss measures to mitigate any excessive inflammation or scarring that might cause a failure after the second attempt.

The various other options to have children that are available to the patient are also discussed to include costs, risks, and time to conception. Because so many of our patients had their first reversal attempt with an already older female, and then with the delays of the failed first reversal attempt and now as they contemplate a redo reversal, this conversation is especially valuable. We also emphasize the importance of close and regular monitoring of the post-reversal semen analysis so that if we do see changes suggestive of obstruction, we can initiate countermeasure to include aggressive anti-inflammatory medications.

Value of Prior Operative Note

The purpose of obtaining the operative note from the first reversal attempt is to help identify any possible challenges or dilemmas and offer any insights that might help with the redo reversal. An ideal operative note from the first reversal should include information to include the location of the vasal defect and repair, anatomic findings, and length of gap. The op note should describe the presence, number, and size of sperm granulomas, whether the scarred vasal segment was excised or bypassed, the gross and microscopic vasal fluid findings, anastomotic technique with sutures used, and intra-op challenges or complications. Unfortunately, this is rarely the case. When performing a redo reversal, it is our philosophy to both accept the outside operative note as accurate and also to assume that there is a possibility that the information is incorrect, possibly as transcription/dictation error, the use of a standardized template, a mistake, or sadly even deliberately misleading to justify a vasovasostomy when in fact no sperm were seen and a vasoepididymostomy was indicated.

Over the years performing many hundreds of redo reversals, there are a number of problems we have seen consistently with outside operative notes. Many doctors today use an abbreviated one-page photocopied template operative note that is the same for every reversal with a few "fill in the blanks." These generic summary notes usually lack any specific information or relevant details. In our experience, what limited information that was provided often does not reflect the reality of what we found at the time of the redo reversal. In our own review of 222 outside redo reversals, we analyzed the vasal fluid and compared the fluid findings to what should have been expected, based on what was described in the operative record and the timing from the first reversal attempt. This suggested that for 1/3 of these patients, the outside operative note most likely did not accurately describe the vasal fluid findings and so the wrong technique was performed on one or both sides [10]. The dilemma is that the written surgical record relies on the surgeon's honesty to describe if they actually looked at the fluid microscopically and if they did, to truthfully describe if sperm were seen as justification to perform a vasovasostomy. We have had patients tell us that the doctor came out after the first reversal and explained that no sperm were seen in the vasal fluid and a VE was probably needed but they did a VV anyway, though the operative note describes the presence of sperm in the vasal fluid. Because of this concern, when we transect the vas at a redo reversal, we analyze the fluid and proceed with the technique based on what we find rather than the vasal fluid findings described in the outside operative record.

Medical Management Pre-redo Reversal

Because of these concerns over probable increased scarring as well as possible unsuspected compromise of a very tenuous vascular supply, it is important to explain to prospective patients that the surgical risks associated with a redo reversal, such as bleeding and atrophy, though still very rare, are higher than with first reversal attempt. Because we assume that the procedure was performed technically well and obstructed as a result of excessive intravasal inflammation, we pretreat our patients with a short course of prednisone. The hope is that these steroids will block any extreme inflammatory response after the redo reversal. These steroids are continued post-op, with the dose and duration based on intraoperative findings and patient health and tolerance.

Redo Findings and Challenges

At the time of the redo reversal, we usually encounter rather dense, vascular scarring in the peri-vasal tissues. This can be localized to just around the vasovasostomy or vasoepididymostomy site or may extend quite a distance along the spermatic cord, which can make finding the prior reversal site an additional challenge. Many times, you may discover only remnants of an atretic scarred vas with a lengthy vasal gap in an already shortened vas where several cm was previously excised. There are occasions when you may encounter the testicle surrounded by thick, desmoplastic scar with the tunica vaginalis obliterated or densely adherent to the underlying testicle or epididymis. This can make just the initial delivery of the testicle and exposing the epididymal tubules a time-consuming challenge.

Compliance with Semen Analyses After a Redo Reversal

We encourage frequent and regular monitoring of the semen analyses to follow sperm counts closely. Close checking the patient's results will allow us, if we see decreasing counts suggestive of excessive intraluminal inflammation, to start pharmacologic intervention during that early window of opportunity and hopefully keep the anastomosis open.

Most would naturally assume that our patients would be more motivated to closely monitor semen analyses after their redo reversal. We have found that the compliance with post-redo reversal semen analyses is minimally better than with their first reversal. To our surprise, we often see long, extended intervals between semen analysis testing after the redo reversal. Many men, even after a redo reversal, are still are not motivated to obtain follow-up sperm counts as directed, well aware how this can negatively impact on outcomes and success. We emphasize before and after the redo, in person, on the phone, by staff, and with written discharge materials the importance of these post-reversal semen analyses to achieve optimum results. Yet many still use the excuses that the testing was inconvenient and embarrassing or they tell us they were busy or simply forgot.

There is an ongoing battle between asking for too many semen analyses or not enough. Frequent sperm counts will provide actionable information, so you can intervene real time with anti-inflammatory medications if the counts are decreasing. Yet if you ask the patient to provide a semen analysis too often, they often become overwhelmed or stressed and stop after providing specimens after one or two. If you have too long an interval between testing, then you lose that window of opportunity to treat when you are best able to reverse any early inflammatory obstruction. We do ask for the patient to provide semen analysis every 4 weeks until stable and well past the timeline when they obstructed after the first reversal attempt.

References

1. Matthews GJ, McGee KE, Goldstein M. Microsurgical reconstruction following failed vasectomy reversal. J Urol. 1997;157:844–6.
2. Hollingsworth MR, Sandlow JI, Schrepferman CG, Brannigan RE, Kolettis PN. Repeat vasectomy reversal yields high success rates. Fertil Steril. 2007;88(1):217–9.
3. Pasqualotto FF, Agarwal A, Srivastava M, Nelson DR, Thomas AJ. Fertility outcome after repeat vasoepididymostomy. J Urol. 1999;162(5):1626–8.
4. Fox M. Failed vasectomy reversal: is a further attempt using microsurgery worthwhile? BJU Int. 2000;86:474–8.

5. Park DW, Kim SW, Paik JS. Microsurgical vasovasostomy following failed vasovasostomy. Korean J Urol. 2001;42:247–53.
6. Paick J-S, Park JY, Park DW, Park K, Son H, Kim SW. Microsurgical vasovasostomy after failed vasovasostomy. J Urol. 2003;169(3):1052–5.
7. Hernandez J, Sabanegh ES. Repeat vasectomy reversal after initial failure: overall results and predictors for success. J Urol. 1999;161:1153–6.
8. Donovan JF Jr, DiBaise M, Sparks AE, Kessler J, Sandlow JI. Comparison of microscopic epididymal sperm aspiration and intracytoplasmic sperm injection/in-vitro fertilization with repeat microscopic reconstruction following vasectomy: is second attempt vas reversal worth the effort. Hum Reprod. 1998;13(2):387–93.
9. Kim SW, Ku JH, Park K, Son H, Paick J-S. A different female partner does not affect the success of second vasectomy reversal. J Androl. 2005;26(1):48–52.
10. Murphy R, Perkins A, Marks MB, Burrows PJ, Marks SF. Post vasectomy reversal semen analysis compliancy. Androl. 2012;33(Suppl 2):42.

Chapter 14
Past and Future Reversal Ideas

Past and Future Vasectomy Reversal Ideas

When sitting at a lecture by a young up-and-coming urologist who was talking about new ideas and advances in vasectomy reversals, a very senior expert sitting next to me leaned over and said "sooner or later everything comes around again. I've seen this before, it will work initially, and everyone will get excited, then over time the numbers will not be what everyone had hoped, and it will be delegated to the back burner until it is reinvented again long after I am gone."

Of course, just because an idea didn't work before does not mean the idea is dead forever. What failed before may come back in the future as a new and improved idea, learning from past failures to create a new technique or advance that propels vasectomy reversal techniques or success to new levels. As the old saying goes, "what was once, will be again." This chapter will briefly cover some of the past attempts to improve reversals that have not been adopted such as laser-assisted reversals, fibrin glue and luminal stents, the concerns over limited microsurgery training in urology residency programs, as well as ideas for future advances with reversals to include robotic-assisted vasectomy reversals, artificial intelligence, and remote reversals.

Laser-Assisted Vasectomy Reversals

In the 1980s and early 1990s, there was a lot of interest with the idea of using the laser for vasovasostomy. The hope was that "spot welding" with a CO_2 or Nd:YAG laser would greatly simplify a technically challenging reversal and allow for faster repair. Though the early animal data was very promising, it became clear that the fusion coagulation of protein on the transected faces of the vas produced significant inflammation. The idea of laser-assisted reversals was abandoned as the outcomes

© Springer Nature Switzerland AG 2019
S. H. F. Marks, *Vasectomy Reversal*,
https://doi.org/10.1007/978-3-030-00455-2_14

were not as good as with the gold standard of hand-sutured microsurgical reversals [1–5]. Variations with an albumin-based solder were also tested [6].

Glue-Assisted Vasovasostomy

As with the use of the laser, the goal with the use of fibrin glue during a vas-to-vas anastomosis was to simplify the technical reversal and allow for faster operative time. Fibrin glue was used with a modified one-layer vasovasostomy using 9–0 nylon sutures hand placed for the inner layer and the outer layer of glue to approximate the outer muscularis layers [7–9]. A recent study at a single center that uses fibrin glue did show that the use of glue did reduce the operative time from 120 min down to 90 min. Though this did result in shorter operative time, the success of 90% for a glue-assisted vasovasostomy is still lower than the 99.5% that can be achieved with a multilayer microsurgical hand-thrown sutures reversal in experienced hands [10].

Intraluminal Stents

There have been two general types of intraluminal stents studied for vasovasostomy with the intended goal to make performing a reversal easier and faster and maintain the patency of the vasal lumen. One approach was to use a solid stent, such as a suture, across the anastomosis to simplify the placement of the intraluminal microsutures. The purpose was to allow for healing of the anastomotic site around the luminal suture and also to prevent the accidental capturing of the back wall of the vasal lumen with subsequent obstruction of the lumen. The second approach was to use a hollow stent to allow for healing with a quicker and less technically challenging repair with passage of sperm through the stent, past the new vasal connection into the abdominal vas [11–18].

There are a number of reasons why stents are still not used today by top experts. In experienced hands, with visualization of passage of the needle and suture with high power magnification, it is very rare to unknowingly catch the back wall of the lumen. Second the success rate with stents was not as high with non-stented reversals. Though temporary solid stents may make passage of the mucosal sutures easier, if left in place, they must exteriorize from the lumen of the vas through a defect through the abdominal vas [19]. When this is removed a short time later, it becomes another source of inflammation and a potential site of mucosal scarring and obstruction. The indwelling absorbable stents made of material such as a chromic suture or polyglycolic acid were also shown to stimulate increased intraluminal inflammation in animal models. One issue with a fixed, hollow stent is that the interwoven muscular layers and the lumen of the vas are not a static tube but rather function as a pump as well as a conduit for the transport of sperm.

The peristaltic waves of vasal muscles contracting propel the sperm up through the vas into the prostatic lumen, while the lumen contracts and dilates as well. Because of this physiologic function of the vas, a stent with no or minimal ability to contract and expand interferes with the needed role of the vas in addition to any increased inflammation [11–19].

Future Ideas, Advances, and Issues with Vasectomy Reversals

The big question is what's the goal – looking for faster, cheaper, better, easier reversals? And at what price? Or is it to provide each and every patient the very highest chances for success so they can achieve their dreams? When looking at new advances in microsurgery and vasectomy reversals, there are several consistent themes that drive innovation. There is always the universal goal of any surgeon to be better and offer higher success for their patients. Then add the desire to be able to modify techniques to perform the surgery faster and so reduce operative time. This allows the surgeon to do more with less and reduce costs to the system and the patient. Advances can also simplify technical aspects of any technically challenging procedure, so it becomes easier to perfect and maintain necessary skills with less time spent on the learning curve. It is important to remember that in our zeal to offer something newer, faster, or cheaper, we must be careful not to compromise patient care or outcomes simply to make the reversal less expensive, easier to perform, or quicker. Why is 80% or 90% success satisfactory when 99.5% can be achieved [20]? I can't imagine anyone that would knowingly tolerate any cardiac, neurosurgery, or joint replacement surgeons who are willing to provide lower success to their patients simply to go faster or reduce costs. It makes sense that advances in our field should at least maintain the quality of care and outcomes with new techniques that improve success.

It is an important for any vasectomy reversal surgeon to understand that when we perform vasectomy reversals, future lives, relationships, and marriages are at stake. It then becomes very clear that settling for "good" results is really not acceptable. Yet looking for ways to go faster or make the reversal easier or cheaper while settling for a lower success seems to be a common theme for many surgeries. An alternative approach might be to instill in all urologists the idea that if they don't perform any procedure, including reversals, often enough to be able to offer the highest level of success, then it is the patient's best interest to refer that patient to an expert that can provide that higher level of care.

Reversal Training Concerns

Many private urologists, urology residency and even some fellowship programs are realizing that they do not provide enough observational and hands-on experience with microsurgical vasectomy reversals. A poster at the 2018 AUA found that most urology residency training directors reported no microsurgical training [21]. At our center we have seen an increase in the number of private practice and academic urologists that have come to watch reversals and some to send their male fertility fellows to us to have a better experience with vasovasostomy and vasoepididymostomy. The number of training options beyond a urology residency or a formal fellowship is very limited. Dr. Phil Li's courses at Cornell in New York City are the only formal microsurgical programs available in addition to those courses taught at society meetings, such as those offered at ASRM annual meetings, currently coordinated by Drs. Peter Chan and Mark Sigman.

Robotic-Assisted Vasectomy Reversals

Robotic-assisted vasectomy reversals are a relatively new idea that seems to be gaining some momentum. At some centers, robotic-assisted reversals are the primary technique for vasectomy reversals. And with future smaller, cheaper, and less expensive robots as well as the use of artificial intelligence (AI)-assisted robotics and advanced haptics to learn and intuitively assist with suture placement, there may be a future role for teaching and performing vasectomy reversals [22].

Clearly the use of a robot is a great option for laparoscopic reconstruction after a pelvic or inguinal vasectomy. Many experts though are still unsure of the advantages for the use of robots in most patients vs. a well-performed standard reversal. Even the robotic gurus will tell you that the use of the robot will not make a poor surgeon into a good surgeon, nor will it make a good surgeon better. The use of robotic-assisted reversals offers one more tool in the urologist's armamentarium for managing the option for pelvic reconstruction of the vas. Another advantage is that the robot eliminates physiologic tremor for those surgeons that have or develop a tremor.

Some other advantages to the use of a robot include improved visualization via multiple angle magnification and the option for additional articulating instrument arms which may eliminate the need for a skilled first assist. Currently, there is much debate as to whether the added acquisition and utilization costs justify the use of the robot when performing vasectomy reversals well by the occasional "reversalist" vs. high-volume surgeons. Simply having access to the robot does not necessarily justify its use [23–34].

Remote Surgery

Because of the limitations of limited access to top experts, there may be a future use for robotics to utilize these advanced technologies to allow for the primary surgeon to be at remote site. Practical applications for the use of robotics early on include military surgery when the surgeon is at remote base from the site of the injury and field hospital. The future may offer top surgeons the option of performing state-of-the-art reversals around the world from the comfort of their primary base facility.

Better Predictors for Success

As we learn more about what aspects of our lives influence our health and fertility, we can better predict which of our patients will have better outcomes from a vasectomy reversal. These may also help us to prepare our patients before their reversal and provide improved after care. This includes understanding the impact of environmental and occupational exposures as well as each individual's genetics that can influence intraoperative decision-making and outcomes. A recent poster by Dr. Jason Hedges and conversations with Dr. Keith Jarvi raise questions about analyzing protein profiles in the vasal fluid to better identify those with patency vs. deeper epididymal obstruction. The future holds many new and exciting ideas for helping our patients to achieve their dream of having their own genetic children after vasectomy [35].

References

1. Lynne CM, Carter M, Morris J, Dew D, Thomsen S, Thomsen C. Laser-assisted vas anastomosis: a preliminary report. Lasers Surg Med. 1983;3(3):261–3.
2. Rosemberg SK, Elson L, Nathan LE Jr. Carbon dioxide laser microsurgical vasovasostomy. Urology. 1985;25(1):53–6.
3. Weiner P, Finkelstein L, Greene CH, DeBias DA. Efficacy of the neodymium:YAG laser in vasovasostomy: a preliminary communication. Lasers Surg Med. 1987;6(6):536–7.
4. Gilbert PT, Beckert R. Laser-assisted vasovasostomy. Lasers Surg Med. 1989;9(1):42–4.
5. Alefelder J, Philipp J, Engelmann UH, Senge T. Stented laser-welded vasovasostomy in the rat: comparison of Nd:YAG and CO2 lasers. J Reconstr Microsurg. 1991;7(4):317–20. discussion 321–2.
6. Trickett RI, Wang D, Maitz P, Lanzetta M, Owen ER. Laser welding of vas deferens in rodents: initial experience with fluid solders. Microsurgery. 1998;18(7):414–8.
7. Ho KL, Witte MN, Bird ET, Hakim S. Fibrin glue assisted 3-suture vasovasostomy. J Urol. 2005;174(4 Pt 1):1360–3. discussion 1363.
8. Busato WF Jr, Marquetti AM, Rocha LC. Comparison of vasovasostomy with conventional microsurgical suture and fibrin adhesive in rats. Int Braz J Urol. 2007;33(6):829–36.
9. Bot GM, Bot KG, Ogunranti JO, Onah JA, Sule AZ, Hassan I, Dung ED. The use of cyanoacrylate in surgical anastomosis: an alternative to microsurgery. J Surg Tech Case Rep. 2010;2(1):44–8.
10. Machen, G, Kleinguetl C, Chen W, Bird E. Vasectomy reversal utilizing fibrin glue reinforcement: one institution's experience. American Society of Andrology and European Academy of Andrology. Andrology, 2018, Supplement, 91. Poster 111.
11. Urry RL, Thompson J, Cockett AT. Vasectomy and vasovasostomy. II. A comparison of two methods of vasovasostomy: silastic versus chromic stents. Fertil Steril. 1976;27(8):945–50.
12. Flam TA, Roth RA, Silverman ML, Gagne RG. Experimental study of hollow, absorbable polyglycolic acid tube as stent for vasovasostomy. Urology. 1989;33(6):490–4.

13. Berger RE, Jessen JW, Patton DL, Bardin ED, Burns MW, Chapman WH. Studies of polyglycolic acid hollow self-retaining vasal stent in vasovasostomy. Fertil Steril. 1989;51(3):504–8.
14. Rothman I, Berger RE, Cummings P, Jessen J, Muller CH, Chapman W. Randomized clinical trial of an absorbable stent for vasectomy reversal. J Urol. 1997;157(5):1697–700.
15. Vrijhof EJ, de Bruïne A, Lycklama à Nijeholt AA, Koole LH. A polymeric mini-stent designed to facilitate the vasectomy reversal operation. A rabbit model study. Biomaterials. 2004;25(4):729–34.
16. Vrijhof EJ, de Bruine A, Zwinderman A, Lycklama à Nijeholt AA, Koole L. New nonabsorbable stent versus a microsurgical procedure for vasectomy reversal: evaluating tissue reactions at the anastomosis in rabbits. Fertil Steril. 2005;84(3):743–8.
17. Safarinejad MR, Lashkari MH, Asgari SA, Farshi A, Babaei AR. Comparison of macroscopic one-layer over number 1 nylon suture vasovasostomy with the standard two-layer microsurgical procedure. Hum Fertil (Camb). 2013;16(3):194–9.
18. Jeon JC, Kwon T, Park S, Park S, Cheon SH, Moon KH. Loupe-assisted Vasovasostomy using a prolene stent: a simpler vasectomy reversal technique. World J Mens Health. 2017;35(2):115–9.
19. Shessel FS, Lynne CM, Politano VA. Use of exteriorized stents in vasovasostomy. Urology. 1981;17(2):163–5.
20. Nyame YA, Babbar P, Almassi N, Polackwich AS, Sabanegh E. Comparative cost-effectiveness analysis of modified 1-layer versus formal 2-layer vasovasostomy technique. J Urol. 2016;195:434–8.
21. Ghayda RA, Bakare T, OHlander S, Pagani R, Niederberger C. Andrology/male infertility subspecialty exposure during U.S. based urology residency training. Poster presented at American Urological Association Annual meeting. San Francisco, California 18 May 2018.
22. Chang KD, Raheem AA, Rha KH. Novel robotic systems and future directions. Indian J Urol. 2018;34(2):110–4.
23. Nagler HM, Belletete BA, Gerber E, et al. Laparoscopic retrieval of retroperitoneal vas deferens in vasovasostomy for postinguinal herniorrhaphy obstructive azoospermia. Fertil Steril. 2005;83:1842.
24. Matsuda T, Muguruma K, Hiura Y, et al. Seminal tract obstruction cause by childhood inguinal herniorrhaphy: results of microsurgical reanastomosis. J Urol. 1998;159:837–40.
25. Pasqualotto FF, Pasqualotto EB, Agarwal A, et al. Results of microsurgical anastomosis in men with seminal tract obstruction due to inguinal herniorrhaphy. Rev Hosp Clin Fac Med Sao Paulo. 2003;58:305–9.
26. Kramer WC, Meacham RB. Vasal reconstruction above the internal inguinal ring: what are the options? J Androl. 2006;27:481–2.
27. Buch JP, Woods T. Retroperitoneal mobilization of the vas deferens in the complex vasovasostomy. Fertil Steril. 1990;54:931–3.
28. Kim A, Shin D, Martin TV, et al. Laparoscopic mobilization of the retroperitoneal vas deferens for microscopic inguinal vasovasostomy. J Urol. 2004;172:1948–9.
29. Etafy M, Gudeloglu A, Brahmbhatt JV, Parekattil SJ. Review of the role of robotic surgery in male infertility. Arab J Urol. 2017;16(1):148–56.
30. Lotan Y. Is robotic surgery cost-effective: no. Curr Opin Urol. 2012;22(1):66–9.
31. Liberman D, Trinh QD, Jeldres C, Zorn KC. Is robotic surgery cost-effective: yes. Curr Opin Urol. 2012;22(1):61–5.
32. Parekattil SJ, Gudeloglu A, Brahmbhatt J, Wharton J, Priola KB. Robotic assisted versus pure microsurgical vasectomy reversal: technique and prospective database control trial. J Reconstr Microsurg. 2012;28(7):435–44.
33. Kavoussi PK. Commentary on "validation of robot-assisted vasectomy reversal". Asian J Androl. 2015;17(2):333.
34. Sangkum P, Yafi FA, Hellstrom WJG. Commentary on "validation of robot-assisted vasectomy reversal". Asian J Androl. 2015;17(2):332.
35. Saitz T, Acevedo AM, Bash J, Cunliffe J, Kilmek J, Ostrowksi K, Fuchs E, David L, Hedges, J. Vasal protein profile and microscopic sperm presence at time of vasectomy reversal. Poster presented at American Urological Association Annual meeting. San Francisco, California 18 May 2018.

Appendix 1. Instruments and Microsutures

This Appendix includes lists of some of the microsutures, microinstruments, regular instruments, and disposable items referenced throughout this book. These are provided as many doctors ask what I use and prefer. Using this list is a good place to start if you don't already have your own microinstruments. Over time, you will decide on what instruments and sutures work best for you. Based on where you practice and any limitations from the institution or facility, some of the items listed may not be available to you.

Microsurgical Instruments

This is a list of the specific instruments that we use and have found to be consistently high quality with good vendor support. The instruments that are best for you will vary from surgeon to surgeon. It is always best to try various instruments from a number of vendors to find the ones that you prefer for your own tray. Ask the sale reps to meet with you and show you the options so you can look at and handle the instruments to be sure that they are exactly what you want and fit your needs. You can also look at and handle microinstruments at various society meetings, such as the annual AUA conference. When you are considering microinstruments, don't think about the cost of each instrument or set but instead consider them to be a long-term investment. The higher-quality instruments are a better value as they are more precise and will do a better job and generally last longer. Be wary of cheap, inexpensive "copycat" instruments as they often break easily or have a short lifespan. For critical instruments, it is smart to have backup instruments just in case one breaks or is damaged (the "two is one, one is none" philosophy). Be sure that whomever cares for these instruments in your practice takes the time to wash and sterilize your delicate microsurgical instruments separately from all the other instruments to prevent inadvertent damage to the tips (Fig. A1.1).

© Springer Nature Switzerland AG 2019
S. H. F. Marks, *Vasectomy Reversal*,
https://doi.org/10.1007/978-3-030-00455-2

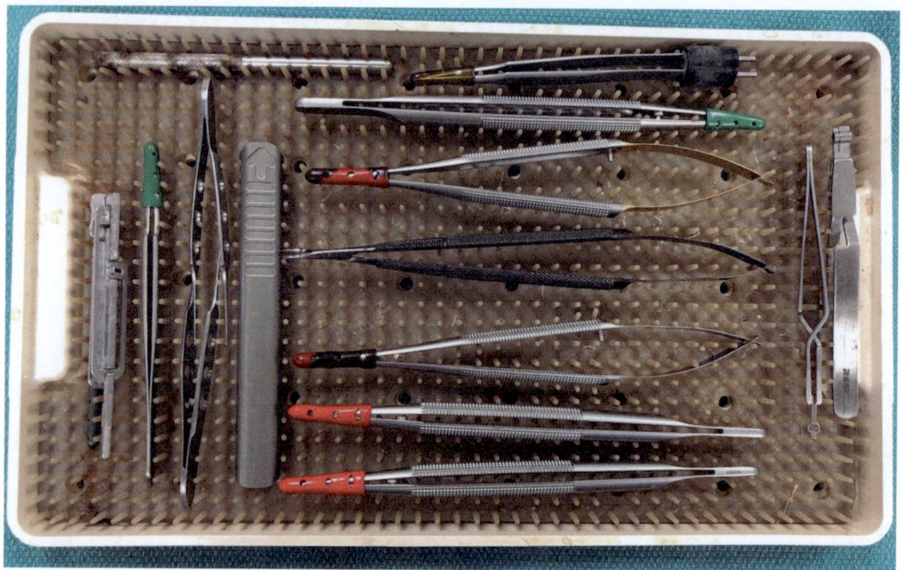

Fig. A1.1 Microinstrument tray. (Photo Credit: Sheldon Marks)

Premade Microinstrument Trays

Below are three preset microinstrument trays from ASSI. These are good "starters" if you perform reversals, though you will have to supplement any premade set with a number of additional instruments. I prefer to create my own trays as some of the instruments in these preset trays are not what I prefer. For example, they provide the 90-degree vas cutting forceps rather than the newer angled vas cutting forceps that offer a higher success. ASSI has created a basic "essentials only" tray (Fig. A1.2), a mid-level set (Fig. A1.3), and a more advanced tray with most of the microinstruments that you would need (Fig. A1.4).

Master List

This is a master list of the instruments, microsurgical and regular, for vasovasostomy and vasoepididymostomy, with additional items you would need on the Mayo stand (Fig. A1.5).

Microinstrument List

Microforceps, round handled, long with tying platform, straight tip (#2) (ASSI.227) (Fig. A1.6.).

Fig. A1.2 Basic microinstrument set (ASSI. GVAS1). (Photo Credit: Accurate Surgical and Scientific Instruments, Corp. [ASSI])

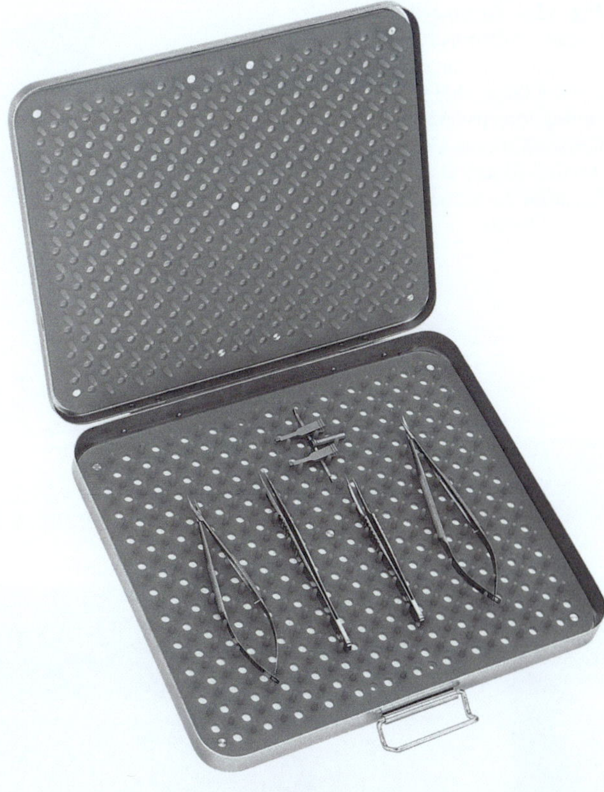

Fig. A1.3 Intermediate microinstrument set, with only the straight and not the angled vas cutting forceps (ASSI.LVAS1). (Photo Credit: Accurate Surgical and Scientific Instruments, Corp. [ASSI])

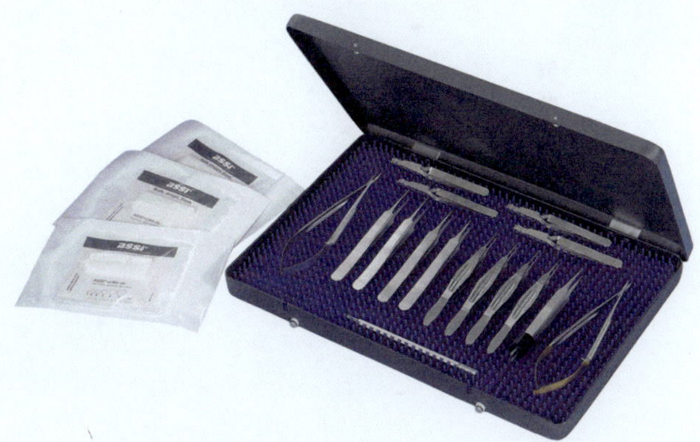

Microtip needle holders, 13 cm, curved microtip, not locking, round handles for 70 and 100 micron needles on the 10-0 and 9-0 suture (ASSI B138).

Castroviejo needle holder, curved microtip, not locking, round handles for 7-0 needles.

Fig. A1.4 Advanced (deluxe) microinstrument tray, with only the straight and not the angled vas cutting forceps (ASSI. GVAS2). (Photo Credit: Accurate Surgical and Scientific Instruments, Corp. [ASSI])

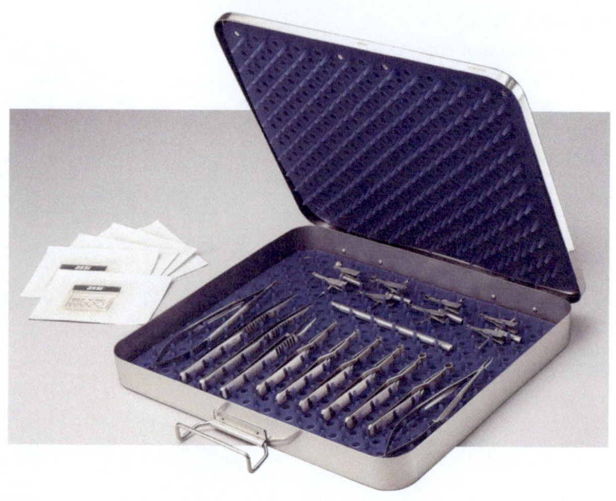

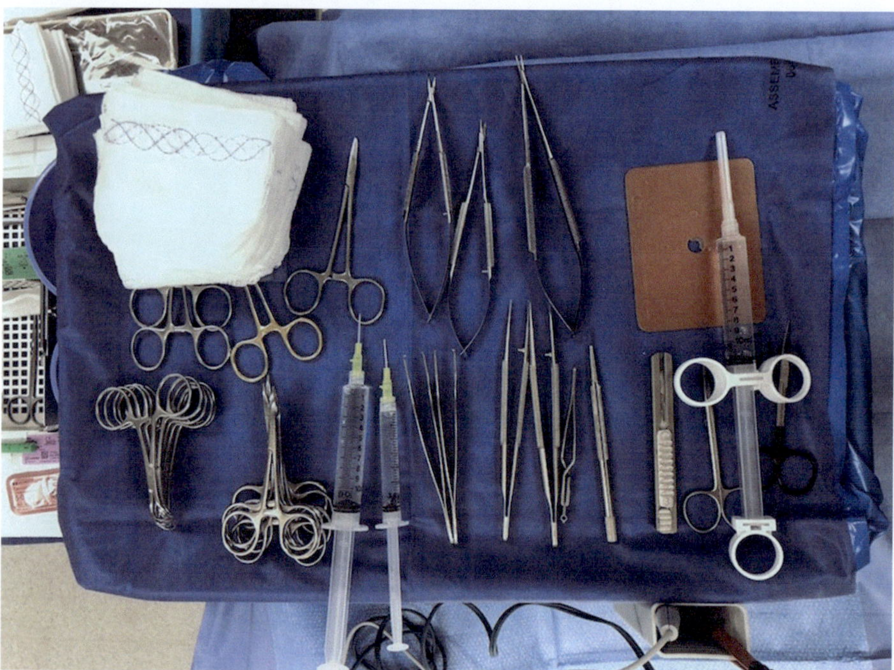

Fig. A1.5 Mayo tray set up with microinstruments and regular instruments, local anesthetic, and irrigation. (Photo Credit: Sheldon Marks)

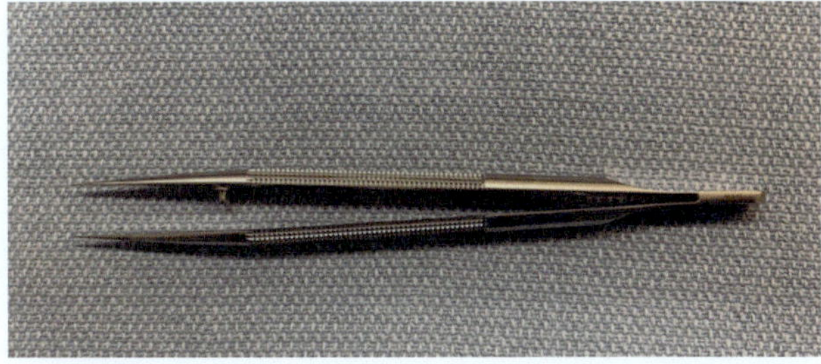

Fig. A1.6 Microforceps with tying platform (ASSI.227). (Photo Credit: Accurate Surgical and Scientific Instruments, Corp. [ASSI])

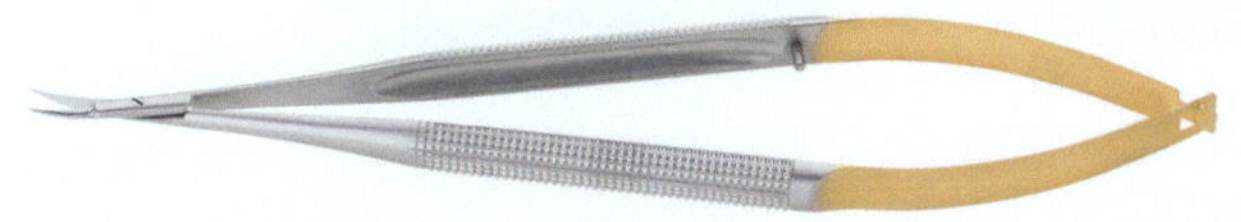

Fig. A1.7 Lipshultz microepididymal scissors (ASSI-SDC15RVL). (Photo Credit: Accurate Surgical and Scientific Instruments, Corp. [ASSI])

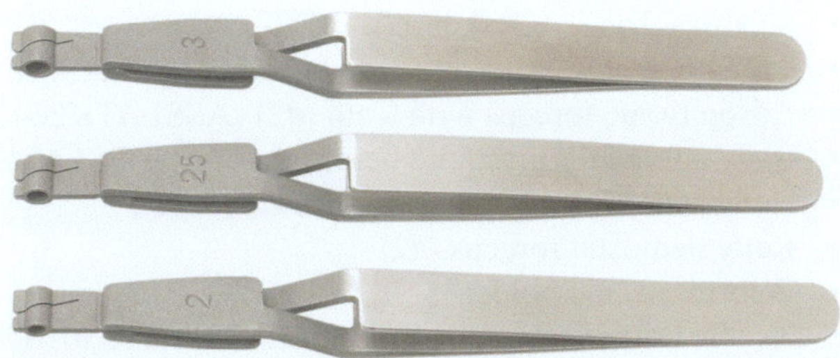

Fig. A1.8 Marks angled vas cutting forceps (Marks Vas ASSI-NHF 2.5, 2.5.15, 3.15). (Photo Credit: Accurate Surgical and Scientific Instruments, Corp. [ASSI])

Lipshultz microepididymal tissue scissors, for incising the tunica over epididymal tubules or creating epididymal windows (ASSI-SDC15RVL). When these scissors become dull or the tips are bent, they can be repaired and be used as microsuture scissors (Fig. A1.7).

Suture cutting microscissors, for cutting 9-0 and 10-0 sutures, which are more durable than the delicate microepididymal scissors (ASSI.SAS15).

Microbipolar, fine and micro, straight pointed tip, 0.25 mm tip diameter jeweler's bipolar forceps, nonstick Noble metal (#2) (ASSI.BPNS11223).

Marks angled vas cutting forceps in 2.0, 2.5, and 3.0 mm (ASSI-NHF 2.5, 2.5.15, 3.15) (Fig. A1.8).

Right-angle vas cutting forceps (3 sizes) (ASSI-NHF2.5, 3.0, and 3.5) (Fig. A1.9).

Microblade holder Denis (BHS11) with straight microblades (CBS35) (Fig. A1.10).

Jeweler's forceps #5, (#2).

Bishop tissue forceps, with teeth (#2).

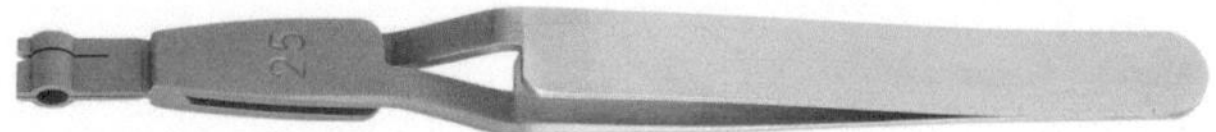

Fig. A1.9 Right-angle vas holding forceps (ASSI-NHF2.5). (Photo Credit: Accurate Surgical and Scientific Instruments, Corp. [ASSI])

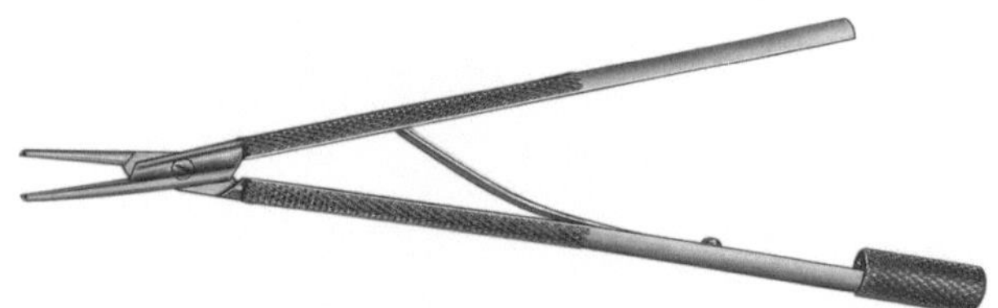

Fig. A1.10 Microblade holder (ASSI-BHS12). (Photo Credit: Accurate Surgical and Scientific Instruments, Corp. [ASSI])

Regular Instruments

- Scissor – Iris (ASSI.A4502)
- Iris Supercut scissors, curved, delicate (ASSI.ASIM 12-0003).
- Adson tissue forceps with teeth (#2) (ASSI.ATK26426)
- Baby curved tip mosquito hemostats (#8) (ASSI 4943)
- Hemostat – fine tip, curved (Miltex 17-002).
- Kelly hemostat forceps (#2)
- Webster needle holder
- Needle holder, silver, smooth jaw (ASSI.ATK 30509-13).
- Allis baby tissue clamp, 6 inch (#2) (ASSI.AG 1227326)
- Backhaus towel clamps (#8) (ASSI.49786)
- Retractors – Senn, sharp or dull, for lifting skin when replacing testicle (#3) (Miltex 11-80/ 11-81).
- Medicine glass, 40 cc
- Safety Scalpel Knife Handle (V. Muller SU 1403-001).
- Needle tip cautery electrode

Microsutures and Disposable Products

Below is a list of the microneedles and other products that we have found at this time to be the best for vasovasostomy and vasoepididymostomy. Over the years we have tried many other needles from a variety of vendors, and these are the specific needles and sutures that we prefer. As with any product, we will continue to consider alternatives that are the same quality but less expensive or ones that are better at the same costs. It is not wise nor is it in the patient's best interest to use cheaper products, as they often result in more microsurgical trauma to the delicate tissues and so increased risks for scarring.

Vasovasostomy Inner Mucosal Layer
10-0 **AA-2334** 6 inch/15 cm black monofilament nylon bicurve M.E.T.$_{TM}$ 100 micron 95°/107° double-armed needles by Sharpoint $_{TM}$.

Vasoepididymostomy Inner Mucosal-Tubule Layer
10-0 **AA-2492** 1 inch/2.5 cm black monofilament nylon bicurve M.E.T.$_{TM}$ 70 micron needle 95°/107° double-armed needles by Sharpoint $_{TM}$

Muscularis Layer
9-0 **AA-1825** 5 inch/13 cm black monofilament nylon ½ circle 149-degree vas cutting 100 micron needle single-armed needle by Sharpoint $_{TM}$

Outer Adventitial Layer
7-0 **1547G** 18 inch/45 cm black nylon monofilament P-6 reverse cutting 8.0 mm ¼ circle needle by Ethilon $_{TM}$

Subcutaneous Layers
4-0 **G422N** 27 inch/70 cm synthetic absorbable PolySyn $_{TM}$ undyed braided coated polyglycolic acid DSM19 precision reverse cutting 3/8 circle single needle by Sharpoint $_{TM}$

Subcuticular Layer
5-0 Caprosyn$_{TM}$ **SC5689G** 18 inches/45 cm undyed monofilament absorbable P-13 3/8 cutting 13 mm needle by Covidien$_{TM}$

Instrument Wipe
2 mm thick, 8.25 cm × 8.25 cm
   Ivalon by Fabco Surgical Products

Skin Marker
Fine tipped, Devon (KS 77642412)

Back Table and Mayo Stand
Back table setup with three bowls – normal saline or lactated Ringers, 100 cc, in the large bowl, heparinized saline in the medium bowl, and prep solution in the small bowl – and local anesthetic in the glass medicine cup (Fig. A1.11).

Mayo stand with additional items added to instruments, to include a large 10 cc syringe with lactated Ringers for general irrigation; two small 3 cc syringes with heparinized saline (one for right and another for left) for vasal irrigation and to assess abdominal patency, both with 24-gauge Angiocath; and a 10 cc control-top syringe and 27 gauge 1.5 inch needle with local anesthetic.

If banking is an option and we are going to aspirate vasal or epididymal fluid for cryopreservation, or possibly perform testicular sperm extraction (TESE), then we also have a TB syringe primed with HTF with a 24-gauge Angiocath and a sterile plastic test tube also with 0.5 cc HTF ready.

All syringes are individually labeled and all medications and irrigations on the field, Mayo stand, and back table are labeled.

Custom vasectomy reversal pack includes all drapes, gauze sponges, foam eye spears, bowls, syringes, and micropens.

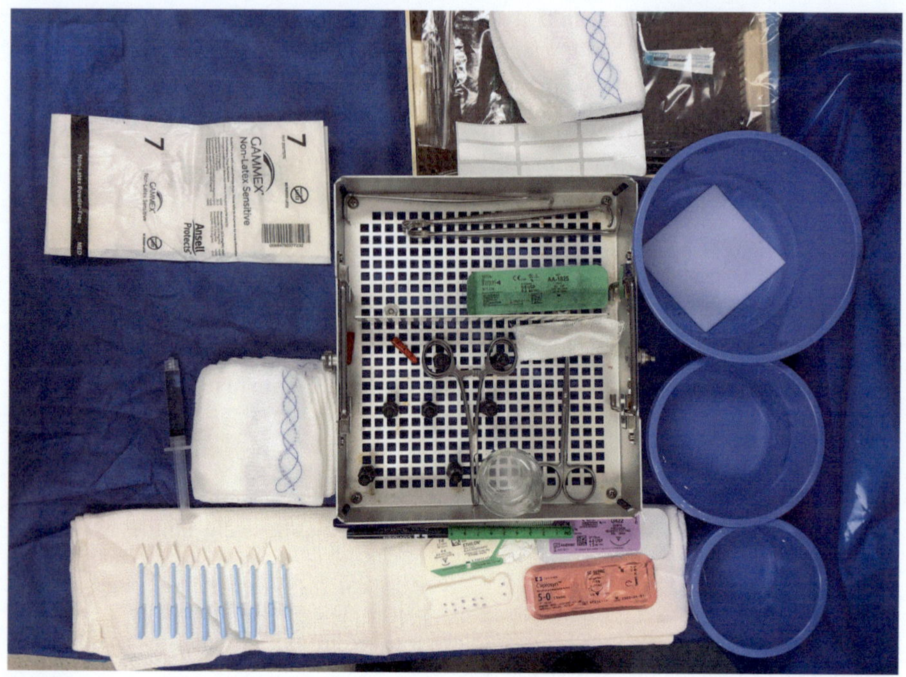

Fig. A1.11 Adjacent back table setup. (Photo Credit: Sheldon Marks)

Instrument wipe (seen in LR solution) is then cut into ¾/¼ section, with the ¾ section for wiping blades and instruments, and then the ¼ portion is cut in ½ with each half perforated with two holes to secure the vas.

ASSI or other straight microblade (cut in ½, flip after first side, hold the second half if needed).

Skin markers (2) – one microtip marker for the microdots and to define the luminal mucosa and a regular tip pen used to ink the arch of the epididymal tubules.

Appendix 2. Resources for the Reversal Surgeon: Androlog, SMRU Discussion Group, Specialty Societies, and Vendors

As part of your ongoing commitment to improve your surgical skills, expand your field of knowledge, and stay up-to-date on current advances and issues in the field of urologic microsurgery and fertility, it makes sense to be an active member of our shared online discussion boards, the new and improved Androlog, as well as the SMRU Discussion Group. In addition, membership in a number of key specialty societies and regular attendance at annual meetings will give you an opportunity to interact and meet with the world's top experts and thought leaders in male reproductive medicine and microsurgery. Below is information on how to become a member of Androlog, the SMRU Discussion Board, and a list of some of the top specialty societies in the USA which are relevant to vasectomy reversals and male fertility. Of course, there are many more societies that you can join in the USA and internationally, often specific for your own country, language, or region of the world.

Androlog

For many years Andrology has been the primary on line moderated discussion forum for more than 1700 of the world's top specialists in male reproductive medicine and surgery. Developed in 1994 and overseen by Dr. Craig Niederberger and his team, Androlog has always been the "go to" real-time resource for sharing information, asking about patient questions, offering your thoughts about clinical problems, or simply reading what others have written. Recently, a new and improved Androlog through Fertility and Sterility has been released.

1. To sign up, register as a member of Fertility and Sterility https://www.fertstertdialog.com/users/sign_up.
2. Then visit the andrology page https://www.fertstertdialog.com/rooms/281-androlog.
3. Then click on the "conversations" tab to read what others have written or to start your own discussion with a question or to review a problem you've encountered.

© Springer Nature Switzerland AG 2019
S. H. F. Marks, *Vasectomy Reversal*,
https://doi.org/10.1007/978-3-030-00455-2

SMRU (Society for Male Reproduction and Urology) Discussion Group
Spearheaded by Dr. Dan Williams, this new online group for SMRU members provides a platform for posting questions or to discuss interesting and challenging cases or problems to the reversal and male fertility community. This forum allows others to reply just to the sender or to the entire group. You do not need to log in to read messages on the SMRU Discussion Group, but ASRM login is required to reply to any posts or start a new discussion.

Society Resources
Information on each of these societies or institutions was taken from their current websites. There may be changes in the information provided since the publication of this book, including contact names, e-mail addresses, websites, or phone numbers so it is best to confirm with their current website if you have any questions or wish to become a member.

Society for the Study of Male Reproduction (SSMR) is the male fertility specialty society affiliated with the American Urological Association (AUA). The SSMR meeting is a half day of relevant and timely presentations held during the AUA annual conference.

- 1100 E Woodfield Road, Suite 350
- Schaumburg IL 60173 USA
- Tel: (847) 517-7225
- Fax: (847) 517-7229
- Email: info@ssmr.org
- Website: ssmr.org

American Urological Association (AUA) is the primary association of urologists in the USA and internationally. The AUA annual international conference, attended by many thousands of urologists from throughout the world, is held every year at a different location in the USA. The AUA has an extensive educational program. In addition, there are many sectional and educational meetings and courses held throughout the year.

- 1000 Corporate Boulevard
- Linthicum, MD 21090
- Toll Free (U.S. only): 1-866-RING AUA (1-866-746-4282)
- Phone: 410-689-3700
- Fax: 410-689-3800
- Website: www.auanet.org
- AUA Membership
- Phone: 410-689-3933
- membership@AUAnet.org

Society for Male Reproduction and Urology (SMRU) is the male fertility specialty society of the American Society for Reproductive Medicine (ASRM), the world's largest fertility society. Membership in ASRM is a requirement for membership in SMRU. The annual meeting is held in conjunction with the annual ASRM international conference held in the USA.

- 1209 Montgomery Highway
- Birmingham, AL 35216-2809
- Telephone: (205) 978-5000
- Fax: (205) 978-5005
- E-mail asrm@asrm.org

Society of Reproductive Surgeons (SRS), also an affiliated society of ASRM, focuses on the surgical aspects of male and female reproductive medicine.

- 1209 Montgomery Hwy
- Birmingham AL 35216
- Phone: 205-978-5000
- email: asrm@asrm.org
- www.reprodsurgery.org

American Society for Reproductive Medicine (ASRM)

The leading society for the advancement of human fertility and reproductive medicine in the USA and internationally, with an annual meeting held in the USA. Though most of the meeting is female fertility focused, there is a large contingent of male reproductive experts that attend and participate in lectures, courses, and of course posters and presentations. ASRM also has extensive educational products.

- 1209 Montgomery Highway
- Birmingham, Alabama 35216-2809
- Telephone: (205) 978-5000
- Fax: (205) 978-5005
- asrm@asrm.org - Main ASRM email address,
- membership@asrm.org - ASRM Membership

The American Society of Andrology (ASA) is a society of clinical, laboratory, and basic science researchers focused on all aspects of male reproductive medicine. The ASA holds a meeting every year in the USA where researchers and clinicians come together to discuss advances in the field.

- Two Woodfield Lake
- 1100 E. Woodfield Road
- Suite 350
- Schaumburg, IL 60173
- Phone: +1 847 619 4909
- FAX: +1 847 517 7229
- E-mail: info@andrologysociety.org

American Association of Tissue Banks (AATB) is the association for anyone involved in sperm banking.

- 8200 Greensboro Drive, Suite 320
- McLean, VA 22102 I
- Phone: 703 827 9582
- www.aatb.org

American Board of Urology (ABU)

This organization oversees continuing urologic education and board certification for urologists.

- American Board of Urology
- 600 Peter Jefferson Parkway
- Suite 150
- Charlottesville, VA 22911
- Phone: (434) 979-0059
- Fax: (434) 979-0266
- www.abu.org

Microsurgery Training in the USA

To improve your microsurgical skills at any point in your career, it is wise to seek out and attend a microsurgical training course. Some are short and a day or more while others may take longer depending on the course specifics. Though there are many microsurgical reversal training programs throughout the world, in the USA there are only two options at this time: the formal courses directed by Dr. Philip Li at Cornell in New York City and ASRM courses at some of the annual meetings throughout the USA, currently directed by Drs. Mark Sigman and Peter Chan. It is smart to be sure that the course you take is taught by top reversal experts with years of extensive, hands-on experience such as these leaders in microsurgery education.

Cornell Microsurgery Training and Research Program

This program offers the only formal institution-based basic and advanced microsurgical training under the direction of Dr. Philip S. Li and the Cornell faculty including Dr. Marc Goldstein and Chair, Dr. Peter Schlegel. This program is part of the Center for Male Reproductive Medicine and Microsurgery in the Cornell Institute for Reproductive Medicine at the New York Presbyterian Hospital-Weill Medical College of Cornell University.

- Phil Li, M.D.
- Professor of Research in Urology and Reproductive Medicine
- Director, Microsurgical Training and Research Program
- 525 East 68th Street
- New York, NY 10065
- (212) 746-5762 or /5768
- E-mail: psli@med.cornell.edu

ASRM Courses

ASRM offers Special Master's Microsurgery Courses some years as part of the annual Congress and Expo conference program. Look at the ASRM meeting program online to see if a course is being taught the upcoming year.

Vendors

These are the vendors and manufacturers that I have found over the years to be a reliable resource for the highest-quality surgical microscopes, specialty instruments, and microsutures to perform vasectomy reversals. Of course, there are many others that you may prefer. I am always eager to learn about new vendors, so I encourage you to contact me with any information on suppliers that you have found to be consistent and reliable with high-quality products. By providing the names of these vendors I am not in any way saying that these are the only resources for many of the products described throughout the book, nor am I vouching for the quality or reliability of the products or delivery. These are simply the ones that I currently use.

ASSI: Accurate Surgical & Scientific Instruments Corporation

Very high-quality microsurgical instruments used by most top reversal experts. They are known for excellent customer service before and after the sale, with reps that have been around for years. You can call them for a catalog or go online. Even better is call and arrange to have their regional representative come out to meet you and discuss what instruments they have to address your needs. We meet with our regional rep at least twice a year in our office.

- 300 Shames Drive, Westbury, NY 11590
- Toll free: 1-800-645-3569
- West Coast Toll Free: 1-800-255-9378

Sharpoint™

Precision microsutures designed, engineered, and manufactured for microsurgical vasovasostomy and vasoepididymostomy. The 70- and 100-micron bicurve needles with MET points are what we have found to be the best.

- Telephone: +1 877.991.1110
- Email: service@surgicalspecialties.com
- 1100 Berkshire Blvd., Suite 308, Wyomissing, PA 19610

Irvine Scientific: USA

HTF (human tubule fluid) Sperm Washing Medium, to maintain sperm quality during sperm retrieval, preparation, and washing procedures.

Catalog ID: 9983Formulation: HEPES-buffered HTF with human serum albumin

- 1830 E. Warner Avenue
- Santa Ana, CA USA 92705-5505
- United States Customer Service/Orders: +1 800 577 6097,
- Phone: +1 949 261 7800
- Fax: +1 949 261 6522

- E-mail: tmrequest@irvinesci.com
- Website: www.irvinesci.com

- Irvine Scientific -Ireland and UK
- Unit 31, Newtown Business Centre, Block D,
- Newtownmountkennedy, Co. Wicklow, Ireland
- Phone: +3 53 1 281 9920
- Fax: +3 53 1 281 9928
- E-mail: irelandoffice@irvinesci.com

- Irvine Scientific - Japan
- 17-35, Niizo Minami 3-chome
- Toda, Saitama 335-0026, Japan
- Phone: +81 48 433 2063
- Fax: +81 48 433 2112
- http://www.isj.jx-group.co.jp

Leica Surgical Microscopes
The highest-quality surgical and laboratory microscopes.

- 1700 Leider Lane
- Buffalo Grove, IL 60089 United States
- 1 (800) 248 0123
- Fax: +1 847-236-3009

Zeiss Surgical Microscopes
Also, the highest-qualitysurgical and laboratory microscopes.

- 1 (800) 442-4020
- Zeiss.com

Prescott's Surgical Microscopes
New and refurbished high-quality surgical microscope sales, parts and accessories, international service, and repair.

- 18940 Microscope Way
- Monument, Colorado 80132
- 1-800-438-3937
- 719-488-2268 Fax
- prescott@surgicalmicroscopes.com
- www.surgicalmicroscopes.com

Index

© Springer Nature Switzerland AG 2019

S. H. F. Marks, *Vasectomy Reversal*,

https://doi.org/10.1007/978-3-030-00455-2